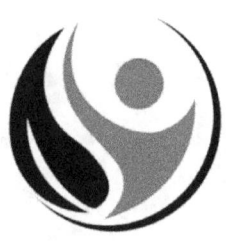

TOTAL MALE

Save Your Life by Taking Charge
of Your Sexual Health

Mark Weis, MD

Douglas Ginter

TOTAL MALE

Save Your Life by Taking Charge of Your Sexual Health

So then, to every man his chance—to every man, regardless of his birth, his shining, golden opportunity—to every man the right to live, to work, to be himself, and to become whatever thing his manhood and his vision can combine to make him.

—Thomas Wolfe

If there's one thing my career as a physician has taught me, it's that smoking is bad for you. Smokers are not bad people, but smoking does bad things to people. The best thing a smoker can do—more than exercise, fitness, healthy diet, you name it—to improve their health is stop smoking. Just as it is undeniable that the #1 cause of death is birth, the #1 cause of male sexual health issues is cigarette smoking.

—Mark Weis, MD

I dedicate this book to my family. To my wonderful father who died at 55 from prostate cancer, my loving mother at 65 from diabetes related problems, my talented younger brother at 35 from internal demons, and my baby sister at 52 from congestive heart failure. All their untimely passings resulted from the unfortunate combination of their not taking responsibility for their own health and the failure of our current health system to recognize and provide effective treatment for their conditions.

I hope the information in the *Total Male* book series helps to make everyone more aware of their potential personal health issues and the easy ways to address them. You have options and nobody can take charge of your health like yourself!

Best wishes to everyone,
—Douglas Ginter

CONTENTS

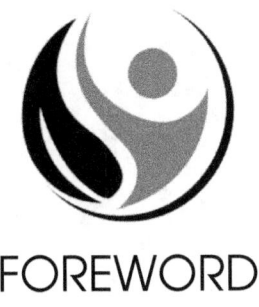

FOREWORD

A fter reading *Total Male: Save Your Life By Taking Charge Of Your Sexual Health* for the first time, I rejoiced to see Dr. Weis plainly describe what modern medicine has recently rediscovered: Sexual health is a useful gauge and guide to *overall health and wellness*. The excellent information in this book should help those who persist in an unfortunate and incorrect morality-based belief that human sexual function is nothing more than physical entertainment. Nothing could be further from the truth!

This first book in the *Total Male series* not only offers clear, step-by-step advice for improving male sexual health; it also explains why knowledge of male sexual health issues can be critical for improving cardiac health, mental health, family relationships, and spirituality.

If you are looking for an effective and easy to understand plan for restoring your *Total Male*, look no further: The information you seek is contained in the pages of this book. I recommend you pay careful attention to its contents, and also make sure that every important man in your life has a copy.

—Charles Runels, MD
Hormone researcher and inventor of Priapus® Shot

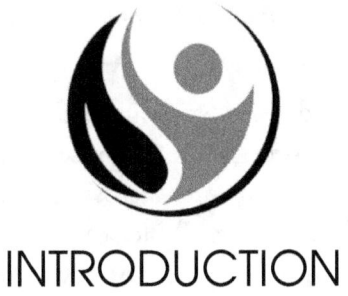

INTRODUCTION

Therefore a man shall leave his father and mother and hold fast to his wife, and the two shall become one flesh.
—Ephesians 5:31

This is book one in a series of health information texts for men. It is for men and about men, and because it is a book for and about men, and men and women walk the road of life together, it is also a book for women. ***Total Male:* Save Your Life by Taking Charge of Your Sexual Health** is important for three groups of readers: (1) Men who want to improve their overall health, sexual health, or quality of life; (2) Women wishing to see the man in their life's improve overall health, sexual health, and quality of life; and (3) Couples wishing to improve their sexual relationship. Men's and women's lives are, and always have been intertwined. No less authority than God himself said:

Let us make man in our image, after our likeness; and let them have dominion over the fish of the sea, and over the fowl of the air, and over the cattle, and over all the earth, and over every creeping thing that creepeth upon the earth.

So God created man in his own image, in the image of God he created him....

Powerful words: words straight from the mouth of the most omnipotent force in the universe. Yet something has gone wrong. Millions of men across the earth—the noble "Man" alluded to in the Bible verse—have plummeted from the lofty position granted by their creator to that of the lowly "creeping thing" mentioned in the same verse.

And why has this happened? Because men lack the information they need to correct the masculine medical problems that lie at the root of their precipitous fall. And why do they lack this information? Because men, noble creatures that supposedly fear nothing—valiant heroes who will wrestle bears, fight lions, swim with sharks, stand in front of a hail of bullets to protect their loved ones, and refuse to shrink from certain death or injury on the battlefield, are afraid to ask about problems with their erectile function, ejaculation, penis size, hormones or prostate. Men, brave warriors in all other aspects of mortal existence, are afraid of doctors and all things medical! Men fear what they don't understand; meaning most would rather remain at home and die from an easily correctable medical problem than go to their physician's office to receive the solution to their problem. And their women— their fair mates charged with watching over and caring for them—allow their men to remain at home, looking on helplessly as their warrior dissolves into a remnant of the man he once was.

Truly a sad state of affairs. Happily, however, there is good news. This travesty can be avoided. Gentlemen, no longer must you suffer in of low self-esteem, your heads hung in shame living lives of social and sexual isolation. Safe and effective solutions to these male sexual health concerns exist. The fall of Man has ended; his rejuvenation has begun. Let's begin an exciting new era ruled by confident men possessing the information that will help them simultaneously overcome their male sexual problems, improve their quality of life, and save them from an early grave!

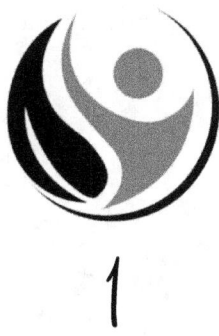

1

Male Anatomy

The penis does not obey the order of its master, who tries to erect or shrink it at will. Instead, the penis erects freely while its master is asleep...The penis must be said to have its own mind, by any stretch of the imagination.
—Leonard Da Vinci (1504)

T he human body is an extraordinary and complicated machine. This machine requires perfect interaction between its billions of cells to accomplish the myriad tasks it performs every day of our lives. Each of these tasks, or biological functions, is a miracle. The fact that our body performs the even greater miracle of effortlessly performing these physical and mental functions that make us human, without our assistance, is beyond mortal comprehension.

Two of these physiological miracles are the male reproductive and urinary systems. These two systems share one organ, the penis, which serves as the literal tip of the spear for the final step in their joint biological processes.

There are 5 steps in the urine formation and release process:

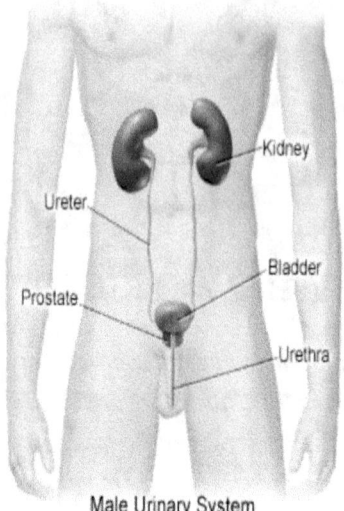

Male Urinary System

1. Blood is delivered to the kidneys where impurities are filtered out and body chemicals adjusted to maintain *homeostasis* (ideal physiological environment).

2. The kidney's filtering process results in urine, which is delivered via the *ureters* to the *bladder*.

3. Urine is stored in the bladder.

4. Urine is voluntarily released from the bladder into the *urethra*, which passes thru the *prostate* gland, located immediately below the bladder, and then enters the penis.

5. Urine is discharged from the penis.

As with the urinary system, the male reproductive system also incorporates the penis in its final step. However, unlike the urinary system, whose purpose is body purification and *homeostasis* (state where all the body's systems are working well together) via the formation and release of urine, the purpose of the male reproductive system is conception. In order for this to occur, the male must produce and release healthy sperm capable of traveling through the female reproductive tract where they can make contact with an ovum (egg) in the woman's fallopian tubes.

There are 5 steps involved in release of sperm-containing ejaculate:

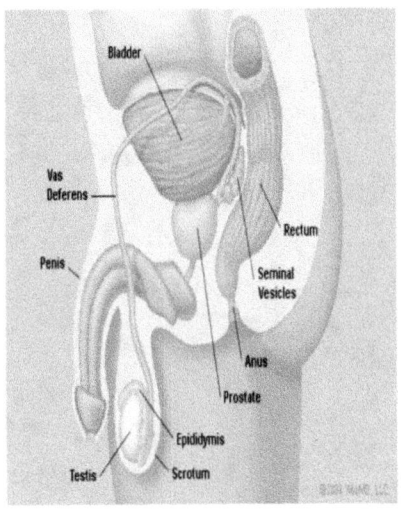

1. Sperm is formed in the *testicles* upon stimulation from the hormones *Follicle Stimulating Hormone* and *Luteinizing Hormone*, both of which are produced by the *pituitary gland* located in the brain.

2. Sperm is transferred to the *epididymis* where it matures.

3. The epididymis transports the sperm via the *vas deferens* to the paired *seminal vesicles* located

underneath and behind the bladder, and just above the prostate gland.

4. The function of the *prostate* gland, a chestnut-sized organ located just below the bladder, is contributing fluids for *semen,* the fluid in which sperm is carried.

5. Sperm-containing semen is released. This final step utilizes the common pathway also used by the urinary system, the *urethra,* which passes through the penis. This fluid is then expelled (*ejaculation*) from the tip of the penis.

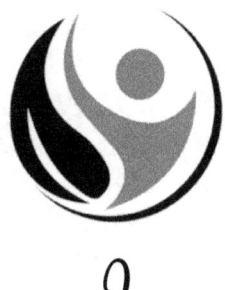

⅔

For Whom The Bell Tolls

*Perchance he for whom this bell tolls may be so ill, as that he
knows not it tolls for him.*
—John Donne

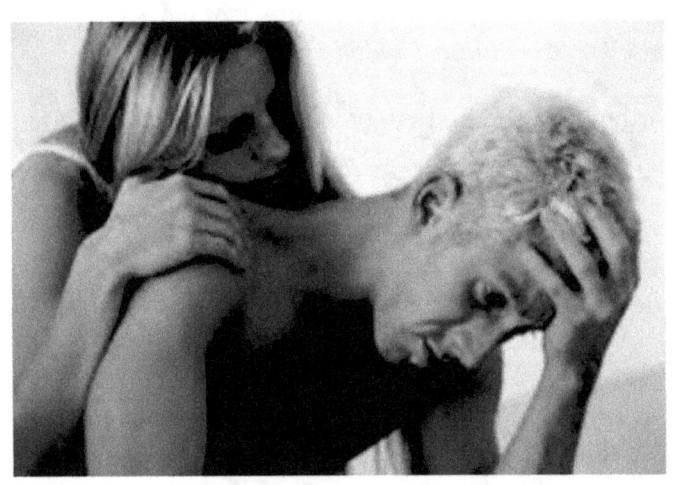

MENKIND: A Play in 4 Acts
By I. M. Manleigh

Act 1

8:00 a.m., Monday

Setting: A small room containing a coffee table and three chairs in the physician's lounge of a community hospital. Three figures occupy the chairs: The first, ROLAND TENNYSON, is one of the town's most respected cardiologists and is a tall, elegant black male in his mid-fifties dressed in a tailored, expensive suit. The second is a stocky, muscular blonde male urologist in his early forties named ALAN BRAND whose white face and thick forearms are deeply tanned from weekends spent working on his horse ranch. BRAND is dressed in scrubs because he is scheduled to perform a complicated prostate cancer surgery in forty-five minutes. The final member of the group is a plump, pleasant elderly gentleman with a kind face wearing an outfit of wrinkled khaki pants, blue dress shirt and oxford loafers. This universally adored local family physician named SAMUEL WORTHINGTON has roamed the halls of this tightly-knit community hospital for fifty years.

Worthington: "Alan, I've got a question for you because you're a urologist. That makes you the resident expert on kidneys, prostates, and the male sexual apparatus, does it not?"

Brand: "That's what my wall of diplomas would suggest, Sam. What's the mystery?"

Worthington: "What's the connection between bathtubs and erection pills? Why do the commercials for that ED drug end with a scene of a bathtub? I know I'm just an ignorant old country doctor and not as sharp as you specialists, but I just can't get my feeble old dinosaur brain around the bathtub thing."

Brand: "Good question, Sam. People ask me about that all the time. You may be old, but you're certainly not stupid. Keeping with that thought, we specialists don't like to advertise this little this tidbit so I'd prefer if you kept it

12

yourself. Most of us believe the hardest job in medicine has to be that of the family doc. You guys must be prepared to deal with any of the tens of thousands of possible medical diseases or situations at every second of every day. How you do that is beyond me. So hats off to you and your generalist colleagues!

"Anyhow, the bathtub thing also baffles me, which makes me think that that bizarre little ending of those ads was probably the result of a 50 cent bet between an advertising executive and a pharmaceutical industry big shot where the advertising guy bet the other fellow he could toss a random thing into the commercials that was so out of step with what they were selling that it would result in people remembering the product better than if they did something that made sense."

Tennyson: "Well, if that was their goal," he laughs, "it succeeded, because look what we're discussing right now!" *He takes a drink from his cup of coffee then continues:* "Hey, have you guys seen the latest stuff on ED and the increased risks it poses for heart attacks and strokes and other vascular disease?"

Worthington: "No, what's the word?"

Tennyson: "It basically says that ED, or erectile dysfunction, is one of the most clear-cut warning signs we have for heart disease. In certain age groups, ED looks like a better predictor of heart attack and, therefore, stroke and similarly potentially catastrophic events, than things like smoking, obesity, family history of heart disease, and cholesterol problems. What's more, if that same person has diabetes, he needed to be in my office yesterday!

13

Brand: "Yeah, I remember hearing about that. And wasn't the most surprising finding the ages of the patients with ED who had heart attacks and strokes?"

Tennyson: "That's correct. The most striking findings were in younger men: men with ED in their twenties and thirties had the highest risk increase, and men in their forties with ED had risks up to fifty times higher than men that age without ED! If you think about the physiology of erection this correlation makes perfect sense because erections result from of a series of events culminating in increased blood flow to the penis. Things like blood vessel disease, or anything else that might hinder blood flow could impair that process. In essence, what ED may be telling us is that the person with it may have atherosclerosis—aka 'hardening of the arteries'—and if atherosclerosis is present in the arteries providing blood to the penis, you'll probably also find it in the in arteries serving the heart, brain and other important organs!"

Brand: "So you're saying ED may actually be a good thing because it can act as an alarm signaling the man who has it that he may have cardiovascular disease and is on his way to a heart attack or stroke? And that if he listens to that alarm and responds quickly he can probably prevent that from happening?"

Tennyson: "Exactly! What this means is that we've got to start re-educating men about ED. Not only must we teach them what erectile dysfunction is and provide them treatments for it, we also must let them know that it may be signaling them that they should get checked out immediately to make sure they don't have a silent and potentially very serious problem brewing."

Brand: "Fortunately, there are now many effective and safe treatments for men who suffer from ED that are not named Cialis®, Viagra®, and Levitra®. Most folks mistakenly believe that if one of those magic man pills doesn't do the trick, or help as much as they'd like it to then they are out of luck. This isn't the truth.

Worthington: *Checks his watch then looks up.* "Well, this has been very informative. If such treatments do exist, then I need to learn about them so I can inform my patients! And while we're at it, I want to learn more about this ED and heart attack risk stuff. Since ED is such a common problem, it sounds like my practice probably contains a large number of middle-aged male patients who at this very moment are working on their first heart attack. I've got to get the word out, so I can find out who they are and prevent that disaster from happening!"

Brand: *Turns to Tennyson.* "You know, Walter, once we start putting out the word about ED and its association with other health risks we are likely to need a cardiologist to send these folks to for evaluation. If I were you, I think I'd go out to my garage tonight and find a hammer and nails because you may need to build a bigger waiting room!"

———————

Impotence. The mere thought of this universally despised word sends shivers down the spine of all men. Dictionary definitions read: "not potent: lacking in power, strength, or vigor; see helpless" and "unable to engage in sexual intercourse because of an inability to have and maintain an erection". No man wants either of these definitions associated with him, because they stand in direct contrast to what society says a man must be: A strong and

15

powerful leader who fathers children, provides for and protects his family, and inspires desire in and sexually satisfies his mate.

What, then, is a man to do who suffers from erectile dysfunction, aka *ED*? Accept the social scarlet letter of permanent affliction that accompanies the dreaded condition? Should he lower his head in shame, avoid social contact and possible sexual intimacy, and live out the rest of his days in a existence of loneliness and quiet desperation? Must the remainder of his life be plagued by a problem that elicits such an intense emotional response, that the scientific community not only made the decision to officially eliminate the word *impotence* from its professional vocabulary and replace it with the term *erectile dysfunction*, they also changed its official definition to the softer (no pun intended!) and kinder phrase: "An inability of the male to achieve an erect penis as part of the multifaceted process of male sexual function."?

The answer to this question is a resounding "Absolutely not!" Fortunately, we now have numerous safe, convenient and effective treatment options for ED. Unfortunately, public awareness of all but a few of them is very low. This is leaving millions of men with ED untreated and unnecessarily suffering the cruel ravages of low self-esteem, relationship intimacy difficulties, and loneliness. If they knew of these treatment options, many of these men could receive effective treatment for this condition!

ED is a very common problem and affects men of all ages. Most men experience occasional erectile difficulty, but for some it becomes a regular and more severe problem. ED can cause low self-esteem, performance anxiety, depression and stress. Understandably, its prevalence increases as men age, but it also affects a large number of young and middle-aged men. There are 33 million ED sufferers in the US, including 18% of men over age 20, up to 39% percent of 40 year-old men, and 50% to 65% of 65 year-old men. Above 70, almost all men experience some difficulty getting or maintaining an erection. Men with ED should find these rates encouraging because it reminds them that they are not alone and have plenty of company. ED rates can be remembered by the following rules: 40% at 40, 67% at 67, and 75% at 75. What's more, male diabetics are unfortunately affected at higher rates and with greater severity than the general population. Put differently, when you go out to eat, shop at a mall, or visit other locations where people gather it's likely that at least one-third of the men around you suffer from ED, and these numbers steadily increase as the group's average age increases.

The problem of ED is not limited to the US. In 1995, the number of ED sufferers worldwide was believed to be 155 million, and this number is expected to more than double by 2025 due to aging of the population. What's more, because of men's inherent reticence to take their ED—or any other—concern to a physician, only one in five men with erectile dysfunction consult a doctor or other healthcare provider. The consequences of this inaction are silently suffering the negative social consequences of ED and vulnerability to the potentially serious health risks accompanying this condition.

The first step in understanding why something doesn't work is learning how it's supposed to work. The penis is an organ containing paired erection chambers called the *corpora cavernosa* which run horizontally down the length of the penis. These chambers are filled with spongy, muscular erectile tissue. Blood flow events leading to relaxation and contraction of these muscular tissues and the penile arteries cause erections to occur and to resolve. Erection, an event regulated by nerves and hormones, is essentially a hydraulic event resulting from blood flow into and out of the penis through the penile artery. Sexual stimulation results in increased blood flow into the penis which leads to trapping and storage of blood within the erectile chambers (corpora cavernosa). This trapped blood results in an increase in pressure and development of *rigidity*, or hardness, of the penis.

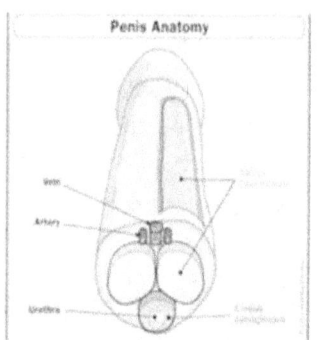
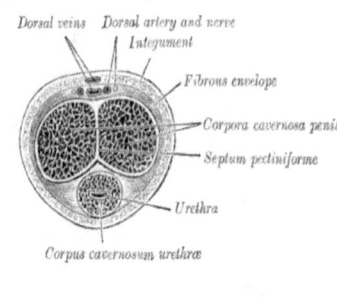

The first step in the chain of events leading to successful penile erection is sexual stimulation. It can be triggered by two differing mechanisms, including (1) direct stimulation of the organ or (2) brain stimulation via fantasy, smells, vision, and numerous other possibilities. Stimulation via either channel results in instantaneous release of chemicals from the brain, which are rapidly transmitted down the spinal cord to nerves in the penis. This causes the blood flow changes that result in erection.

CAUSES OF ERECTILE DYSFUNCTION

There are numerous medical, social or emotional issues that can interfere with this process. For example, anxiety, fear, or mental stress related to partner issues can prevent requisite brain signals from reaching the levels needed to induce erection. Medical conditions such as damaged or blocked blood vessels, and nerve injury from conditions such as diabetes, spinal cord injury, or other neurological illness, can prevent the proper blood flow that leads to the trapping of blood needed for successful erection. One analogy many men find helpful when attempting to understand the erectile process is to think about tires. First, a firm, full tire requires a hose that can rapidly deliver a large amount of air into the tire. This air must be immediately trapped inside the tire by a valve that keeps the air within the tire. In our example, the hose represents the arteries that carry the blood into the paired erectile chambers of the penis. The valve mechanism represents the physiologic process that ensures the blood remains trapped inside the erectile bodies until ejaculation occurs or the sexual stimulus has passed.

Again, penile erection results from a process beginning with the man becoming sexually excited (*arousal*). In order for this to occur, his brain must be able to effectively relay, or send, the proper signals to the nerves in his penis. Stimulation of these nerves causes increased blood flow into the penis, with resultant tissue expansion and penis hardening. Therefore, anything that interferes with the nervous system or the blood circulation can cause, or contribute to ED.

ED causes are divided into two major classifications: (1) organic—which means "caused by the body"; and (2) psychogenic—meaning "caused by the mind". *Organic* ED results from physical problems. It is usually gradual in onset (slowly develops over months and years) and includes problems with erection strength, duration, or both. It is very predictable and the most common cause is circulatory problems. Other common organic causes of ED include

19

untreated or poorly treated, longstanding high blood pressure, diabetes, or high cholesterol. These conditions are all known risk factors for circulation problems—especially when a person suffers from more than one of them. One extremely important note: cigarette smoking is the most important independent (by itself) risk factor for ED, and can also cause the other medical conditions mentioned above.

The organic causes of ED are easily remembered by their medical sub-classifications. These four sub-classifications are (1) *Vasculogenic* (Circulatory System): conditions that affect blood flow to the penis; (2) *Neurogenic* (Nervous System): conditions that affect the nervous system (brain, spinal cord, and the nerves that come off the spinal cord that go to the arms, legs and internal organs). Neurogenic conditions/ED causes interfere with transmission of the messages that cause the blood flow changes that lead to erection; (3) *Hormonal* (Endocrine System): medical problems or other conditions that affect levels of the hormones required for erection; and (4) *anatomical*: conditions that affect the physical structure or workings of the penis.

Examples of vasculogenic conditions that can cause ED include cardiovascular diseases such as *atherosclerosis* (hardening of the arteries); high blood pressure; and *diabetes mellitus*, known by most as diabetes. Diabetes, a hormonal disease resulting from underproduction of the hormone insulin, leads to blood sugar imbalance. This condition can cause serious problems with both the penis's blood supply and nerves, so it is also included in the neurogenic conditions category. Diabetes is also included in the hormonal cause category, because it results from a disease caused by a hormone deficiency syndrome. As you can see, diabetes is a huge risk factor for ED and the risk for diabetic smokers is outrageously high.

Neurogenic conditions that can cause ED include spinal cord injuries or neurological disorders, multiple sclerosis, diabetes mellitus, Parkinson's disease, strokes, and other diseases of the nervous system.

Common hormonal causes of ED include (1) *hypogonadism*—a condition also known as low testosterone syndrome and more popularly known as *Low T*, that results from underproduction of the male hormone, testosterone, by the testes; diabetes mellitus; (2) *hyperthyroidism*—a syndrome caused by an overactive thyroid gland; (3) *hypothyroidism*—a syndrome resulting from an underactive thyroid gland; and (4) *Cushing's syndrome*, a complicated and dangerous metabolic syndrome resulting from overproduction of the hormone cortisol.

Finally, any injury, birth defect, scarring or other physical defect of the penis that interferes with the penis' nerve supply or blood flow is considered an anatomical cause of ED. A relatively common example (up to 5% of the male population) of an anatomical ED cause is *Peyronie's disease*, an abnormal curvature of the penis resulting from autoimmune disease that scars the lining of the corpora cavernosa. This irregular curvature of the male sex organ impairs function of the erectile chambers by restricting their ability to perform the blood flow activities required for erection.

The second major classification of ED causes is *psychogenic*. Again, psychogenic means having to do with the mind. The list of psychogenic causes includes mental concerns that interfere with normal transmission of chemical messages from the brain to the nerves in the penis.

This in turn results in the blood flow changes leading to erection. Common psychogenic causes of ED are depression, anxiety, bipolar disorder, schizophrenia, severe work or other life stress, history of sexual abuse, PTSD, performance anxiety associated with prior erectile failures, a new partner, and many others.

Another very common ED cause is medications that interfere with the physical events that must occur in order to achieve effective and sustained erection. An unfortunate result of our medicalized society—especially amongst seniors—is many of us take multiple medications. Tens of thousands of prescriptions are written every day that can contribute to ED. Examples of drugs which—either by themselves or in combination with other drugs or already-existent medical conditions—can cause ED include:

- diuretics used to treat high blood pressure, heart failure and kidney disease

- many types of blood pressure pills such as beta-blockers

- fibrates used to treat high cholesterol

- antipsychotics used to treat mental health conditions such as schizophrenia, bipolar disorder, dementia, treatment-resistant depression, and severe sleep problems

- chemotherapy agents taken by cancer patients

- antidepressants—newer drugs targeting serotonin are extremely common ED offenders due to their widespread use

- corticosteroids used in treating allergy, asthma, autoimmune and severe arthritic disorders, and hormonal imbalance

- H2-blockers such as Cmetidine and Ranitidine used to treat stomach and esophageal disorders

- anti-epilepsy drugs used in seizure disorders and chronic pain management

- antihistamines used for allergic and other conditions

- anti-androgens used in prostate cancer and other conditions

Finally, this lengthy list of ED causes includes lifestyle and behavior items. Examples include excessive alcohol use; excessive tiredness; cigarette smoking; illegal drug use such as cocaine, heroin, and cannabis (marijuana). Many men find that instituting a simple change in their life, such as not drinking alcohol on days they plan to engage in sexual activity, can help reduce or even completely overcome their ED. That being said, the greatest risk by far for developing ED is cigarette smoking. The first step any smoker with ED should take to improve their erectile function is immediate and permanent smoking cessation.

ED TREATMENT OPTIONS

What You Probably Know

The year: 1996. The word: Viagra®. Viagra®: the drug that permanently changed the conversation about ED and men's sexual health. The immense impact of Viagra®, scientific name *Sildafenil*, allowed male sexual health concerns to burst from the box in the attic, where they had been safely confined for generations to land smack dab in the middle of the kitchen table, the family room, and the corporate water cooler. This once-taboo subject which caused men to silently slink from the room for thousands of years, was instantly considered appropriate conversation at cocktail parties, church socials, and—horror of horrors—the marital bedroom! Thank you, Viagra®, for bursting this once-impregnable vault. The box you opened did not contain Pandora; it contained the opportunity men badly needed. You have done the men of the world a great service.

However, friend Viagra®, while you are considered a superhero by tens of millions worldwide, you aren't perfect. You were designed to be a one-size fits-all tool to help men with ED. And while you and your look-alike competitors—Cialis® (*tadalafil*) and Levitra® (*vardenifil*)—have been very helpful, you do have two problems: (1) you don't always work, and (2) on occasion you cause some fairly serious side effects.

Viagra®, Levitra® and Cialis® are scientifically classified as *5-phosphodiesterase inhibitors* because of their effect on an enzyme involved in the stepwise process of penile erection. These drugs aid men with ED by increasing blood flow into the erectile tissue in the penis upon sexual arousal. However, none of these products have any effect on sexual arousal. They only work when a man is sexually aroused, and have no effect on sex drive itself. On that note, any urban legends you might have heard about women using them for purposes of orgasm enhancement are beyond the scope of this book. The mechanism of action, or way that these drugs work, is:

1. After sexual stimulation, the penile erection process begins with release of a chemical called *nitric oxide*.

2. The release of nitric oxide causes blood vessels in the erectile chambers to dilate. This results in their widening and being able to accept an increased amount of blood.

3. The increased blood becomes trapped in the erectile chambers and results in penile erection.

4. Ejaculation causes the valve holding in the trapped blood to relax, allowing the blood to return to the general circulation and loss of erection.

The discovery of these drugs is a result of what medicine calls *serendipity*, which is when a drug being evaluated for one disease or medical issue is accidentally found to work for a completely different problem. In this instance, the compound we know today as Viagra® was being evaluated for its usefulness on high blood pressure and *angina pectoris* (chest pain associated with heart blockage). During these studies, the investigators stumbled onto the fact that it had strong effects on penile erection. Boy, I bet they were surprised! And pleased, because Viagra® has become one of the most profitable drugs in history.

These drugs, called *PDE-5s* by medical practitioners, have helped improve the sex lives of millions of men and their sexual partners. All three drugs work similarly, with their only significant difference being duration of action (Cialis'® erectile potentiating effects generally last longer than those of its competitors). The table below lists these products' doses and time required for them to begin working. As you can see, Levitra® and Viagra® look very similar on paper while Cialis'® dramatically longer duration of action separates it from these two.

Product	Duration of Action	Dosages (mg)	Action (minutes)
Cialis®	36-48 hours	5, 10, 20	Onset: 60-120 Peaks: 120
Levitra®	4-6 hours	25, 50, 100	Onset: 20-30 Peaks: 60
Viagra®	4-6 hours	50, 100	Onset: 20-30 Peaks: 60

Although the PDE-5s have been an incredibly welcome addition to the lives of their men with ED, these drugs have three basic problems: first, they don't work for everybody; second, in the people they do work for, some experience an incomplete, or somewhat unsatisfactory response (their erection is not as hard or doesn't last long enough for them or their partner to have a mutually rewarding and satisfying sexual experience) and last, because of their mechanism of action (relaxing blood vessels), they can cause side effects ranging from mild (headaches, flushing, heartburn, nasal congestion and runny nose) to more severe (vision difficulty, dizziness and fainting spells that can result in injury). The likelihood of dizziness and fainting occurring are more likely if the person drinks alcohol or takes nitrates (nitroglycerin) for heart problems.

Does that mean the PDE-5s are bad things and their list of possible problems outweighs the benefits of using them? Absolutely not! These drugs are both effective and safe if used correctly. During the early years of their use, rumors abounded regarding risk of death with their use. The truth of the situation is that most of the initial users were older men, so it's likely that many of these early users had heart problems. It makes sense that when these men with relatively severe medical problems began engaging in a vigorous activity requiring significant mental stimulation and physical exertion (sex), some would have heart attacks or other medical issues. Imagine the number of emergency department visits that would have resulted had these same sedentary men chosen to start playing racquetball or run wind sprints in their neighborhood instead of chasing their startled wife around the house with their newfound erections! Fortunately, the death risk was unsubstantiated. Long-term studies show the risk of a man dying from using PDE-5s for ED is the same as his dying from an automobile crash.

All that's well and good; however, it would be nice if men suffering from ED had other treatment options which worked well and possessed few side effect concerns. Happily, men are in luck because numerous other effective and safe ED treatment options do exist!

ED TREATMENT OPTIONS

What You Probably Don't Know

Low testosterone syndrome, also known as *Low T*, is a common cause, or significant contributor to ED. This subject is discussed in depth in the next chapter, so is not addressed here.

Alprostadil is a medication that helps facilitate erection by causing blood vessel dilation which increases blood flow to the penis. It can be given either by injection or as a suppository.

The suppository form, brand name MUSE® (Medicated Urethral System for Erection), is given by placing the small suppository (about the size of half a rice grain) into the opening at the tip of the penis. The suppository form is not as effective as the injectable form, resulting in effective erections in 30%-40% of men.

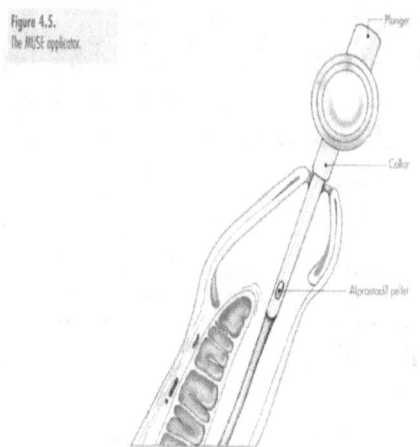

Figure 4.5.
The MUSE applicator.

Plunger

Collar

Alprostadil pellet

The injectable form of Alprostadil, available as brand names Caverject®, Edex®, and Prostin VR®, is given by injecting the medicine directly into the penis. All three of these medicines have identical components; they have different names because they are produced by different companies. These injection methods are all very effective, resulting in erections in 80% of men regardless of ED cause or patient age.

Those of you paying attention may be thinking: Did he just say "shot in the penis?" "Shot"—as in a "sharp needle"—being stuck into the most sensitive part of my body? No way, no how! I don't care how badly I'd like to be sexually active again, ain't nobody sticking a needle into my most valuable and pain-sensitive possession!

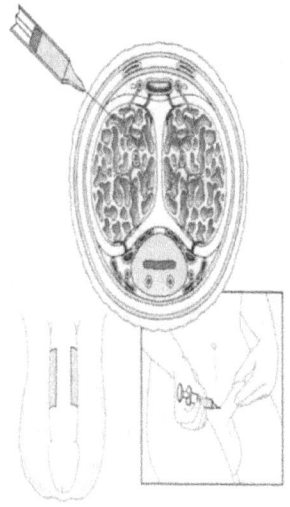

Figure 4.4.
Administration of Caverject. Caverject should be injected into the centre of the corpus cavernosum, avoiding the dorsal neurovascular bundle and ventral urethra.

Reasonable concern. Thankfully, the shot in question is given at the base of the penis (the much-less-sensitive area where it exits the body) and the medicine goes into the erectile chambers. The injection is given by a very tiny diabetic needle and is nearly painless because this area, unlike the extremely sensitive tip of the penis, has very few nerve endings.

While Alprostadil is a relatively effective ED treatment option, it has some mild drawbacks: (1) the window of opportunity for achieving erections via this method is relatively brief (only about 1 hour); (2) use should be limited to three times per week with twenty-four hour breaks between treatments; and (3) men with penile implants, anatomical problems with their penis, disease processes that can impair penile blood flow or who have bleeding disorders such as leukemia, sickle cell disease, and others, should not use it.

Conversely, a positive aspect of Alprostadil treatment is that its effects are fairly predictable, with onset of erection usually occurring within 5-20 minutes of treatment. In addition, some users find their erection may persist after ejaculation, creating the opportunity for continued intercourse—an effect usually appreciated by the most important member of the sexual duet your partner.

Another injectable ED treatment is *Papaverine*. Papaverine, like the Alprostadil-containing products and the PDE-5s (Viagra®, Levitra®, and Cialis®) is also a vasodilator that causes penile blood vessels to expand and accept increased blood flow. Papaverine treatment differs from the well-known PDE-5s, which are pills taken by mouth, in that it is delivered directly to the source of the problem like the other penile injections. Again, when the drug is injected into the erection chamber of the penis, known as the *corpora cavernosa*, the blood vessels dilate and blood flow increases to the penis, resulting in an erection.

Other injection options include *Bi-Mix*—a custom-prepared combination injection incorporating two of the three injectable compounds used for ED treatment (Papaverine, Alprostadil, and Phentolamine), and *Tri-Mix*, which incorporates all three. Note: *Phentolamine* is never given alone because by itself it has little effect on ED, but its presence improves the effectiveness of both Papaverine and Alprostadil.

Vacuum Constriction Devices, or VCDs, are external pumps men with ED can use to get and maintain an erection. A VCD has two components: (1) an acrylic cylinder with a pump that is attached directly to the end of the penis; (2) a constriction ring or band the user places at the base of the penis where it exits the body. The cylinder and pump create a vacuum that causes penile erection by forcing (pulling) blood into the penis. The constricting band maintains the erection by trapping the blood in the erectile chambers that was forced into the penis by the suction. Users of this treatment method, which results in satisfactory erections for 50%-80% of ED sufferers, has some potential drawbacks: (1) penile injury if the device and band are left on for too long; (2) intercourse episodes and erection duration must be limited to no longer than thirty minutes; and (3) as with penile injection treatments, should not be used by men with bleeding disorders.

The *penile implant*, also known as a penis pump, is another very effective ED treatment option. It is usually chosen by men who have had disappointing results with one or more of the therapies described above, or who have been rendered impotent as a complication of urological procedures such as surgeries for prostate cancer or prostate enlargement. Unlike the rigid penile implant, the inflatable pump is a soft, fluid-filled device surgically placed in the erectile chambers of the penis that can expand and contract without losing elasticity. While these mechanical devices provide a solution for surgically injured men, they usually do not provide the same quality of erection seen with erections induced by natural means.

There are two kinds of implantable penis pumps: two-piece and three-piece.

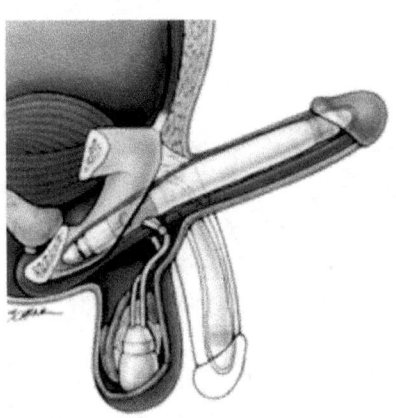

Two-piece Inflatable Penile Implants for erectile dysfunction consist of a pair of fluid-filled cylinders that have reservoirs at the end of each cylinder. The cylinders are implanted into the penis and a tiny pump is implanted in the scrotum. Squeezing the reservoirs implanted in the scrotum forces fluid into the penis which is trapped and results in erection.

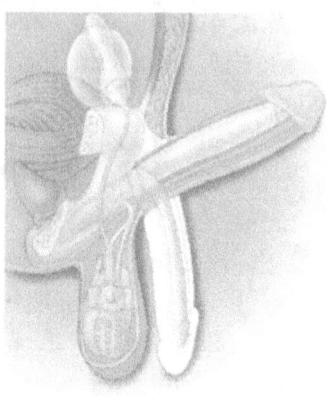

Three-piece Penile Implants include a pair of cylinders, a pump, and a fluid-filled reservoir, the latter of which is implanted in the lower abdomen. This device requires more fluid, thus the addition of the reservoir placed in the abdomen. Its mechanism of action is similar to that of its two-piece cousin.

Both forms of inflatable penile implants work on the same principle as a bicycle pump.

(1) When the man wants to achieve an erection, he pumps up his penis by squeezing and releasing the pump a few times. This forces fluid into the erectile chambers and initiates the erection.

(2) When the erection is no longer desired, he deflates the device by bending the penis (two-piece) or releasing a valve on the pump (three-piece).

The final penile implant option is the *rigid penile implant*. This non-inflatable treatment option consists of semi-rigid rods implanted into the erectile chambers running the length of the penis. When the man is ready for sexual intercourse, he achieves instant erection by lifting the penis, which straightens (locks) the implant. The erection is easily reduced upon completion of sexual activity by bending the rods back to their relaxed position.

The non-inflatable penile implant has some advantages over its inflatable competitor: it is a less complicated surgical procedure, and it tends to be easier to use for men or their partners with manual dexterity issues (no pump to squeeze).

A fairly recent development in the treatment of ED gaining popularity is the *Priapus Shot*™. This safe and effective ED and penis enhancement treatment utilizes *PRP* technology (plasma rich protein) to heal injured or dysfunctional erectile tissue AND improve penis size and cosmetic appearance at the same time! One of the unique advances of using this technology to treat ED is that, unlike the many medications that treat erectile dysfunction by affecting blood flow and therefore facilitating erection, the Priapus Shot™ helps rejuvenate and regenerate penile tissue.

The Priapus Shot™ involves injecting the penis with a substance created from blood known as Platelet Rich Fibrin Matrix (PRFM). PRFM is created via an exciting new medical technology called *Platelet Rich Plasma*, which goes by the moniker *PRP*. PRP is being used to help "heal" or improve a wide diversity of conditions ranging from deteriorating arthritic joints and severe skin injury to penile enhancement.

PRP's mechanism of action is fascinating and has created an aura of excitement among today's forward-thinking healthcare professionals, because it creates nearly-endless possibilities for helping both injured patients and persons that simply want to improve their appearance. Platelets (the "P" in PRP) are components of blood critical to the blood-clotting process. They and other components in human blood migrate immediately to a site of injury where they release a variety of factors that respond to tissue injury which initiate and promote healing. By concentrating platelets at the site of injury (PRP), healthcare providers have the potential to enhance the body's natural capacity for healing.

PRP contains growth factors which stimulate the body to repair and restore tissues using its own natural processes. Since the patient's own blood is used in this procedure, PRP alleviates the risk of allergic reaction or sensitivity. Other than the usual possible risks associated with any procedure, including pain, swelling, and infection there are no known significant risks of using PRP in this way.

UNAPPROVED ED TREATMENTS

Apomorphine (brand name Uprima®) is a drug used in the treatment of Parkinson's disease that acts on dopamine, a brain chemical. It has been approved for treatment of ED in Europe, but is no longer available in the United States because its production was discontinued by its manufacturer.

TREATMENTS THAT DO NOT WORK IN ED

Trazadone is an antidepressant infamous for its extremely rare, but potentially serious side effect of *priapism*, which is a sustained erection requiring surgical intervention to correct. Obviously, Trazadone has no role

34

in the treatment of ED, but is included here with the goal of preventing ED sufferers from erroneously using it for this purpose.

Are you interested in looking better, feeling better, and improving your sex life? Go to **www.totalmale.com** to learn more about ED, premature ejaculation, low testosterone syndrome, prostate health, penis enhancement, other male sexual health issues, increased longevity, and improving your overall quality of life.

For more in-depth information on your hormones, read our book My Hormones; A simple guide to better and longer living, or go our website, **www.myhormones.com**.

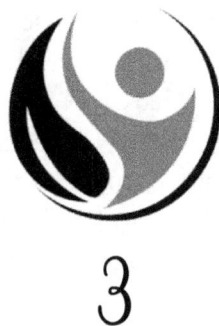

3

Life in the Balance

To acquire balance means to achieve that happy medium between the minimum and the maximum that represent your optimum. The minimum is the least you can get by with. The maximum is the most you're capable of. The optimum is the amount or degree of anything that is most favorable towards the ends you desire.
—Nido Qubein

Saving Menkind

<u>Act 2</u>

12:00 p.m., Tuesday

Setting: The noisy and chaotic hospital cafeteria. Our three characters rendezvoused to continue their male health issues discussion over lunch.

<u>Tennyson</u>: "Thank you, Alan, for referring that nice gentleman with ED to me. I did an EKG on him and it looks like he may indeed have a heart problem. His blood pressure was also a bit high, so I scheduled him for a complete cardiac evaluation later this week. I also whispered in his ear that it wouldn't hurt if he'd stop eating like a college freshman who just discovered the unlimited lunch buffet in his dorm!

On a different note, yesterday we discussed advertising and erection pills and that got me thinking about the increasing number of ads on TV and the Internet about *Low T*. I'm curious as to your take on this, Alan—what with your being our resident gonad specialist."

<u>Brand</u>: *He is amused and chuckles.* "Gonad specialist, huh? Would that make me a *gonadologist*? If so, let's keep that between us, because I seriously doubt a strange title like that will help my street cred! As to your *Low T* question, that's an interesting story. Historically, the diagnosis and treatment of men with testosterone problems has been restricted mostly to the area of infertility, because men with low testosterone levels often produce inadequate or low quality sperm. This can render them unable to father children. Interestingly, though, testosterone has lately become one of the hottest topics on the Internet—not only because of its role in muscular development and sex, but also because of the increased risks for numerous serious medical problems associated with its deficiency."

<u>Worthington</u>: *Instantly alert.* "Medical problems, such as…?"

<u>Brand</u>: "You name it, and it's probably on the list: Heart disease, osteoporosis, hypertension, ED, premature ejaculation, chronic fatigue, insomnia, low sex drive, joint

38

pains, delayed healing from injury, decreased exercise performance, breast enlargement, weight gain, muscle loss, and many more. Why do you think pro athletes take such great risks to get their hands on testosterone and related compounds? Testosterone is the elixir of life, the magic potion that makes the world go 'round. Low T is the worst thing to happen to men since the invention of the vibrator!"

Tennyson: "Did you say heart disease and high blood pressure?"

Brand: "That I did, my friend."

Tennyson: "Whoa, that's news to me! And the rest of that list sounds like it was snatched from a post-apocalyptic horror movie. How come a guy like me who is supposed to be one of the finest cardiologists walking Planet Earth, doesn't know these things?"

Brand: "From what I gather, you're in the majority. This information hasn't found its way to many of our colleagues yet. Regarding low testosterone syndrome, it appears the general public knows more about testosterone than the majority of the medical community. In my opinion that's a disgrace."

Worthington: "Hold on a second there, cowboy! Before you go flinging hormonal stones at our medical brethren, you should stop and consider why this state of affairs likely exists."

Brand: "What is your theory? Enlighten me, please."

Worthington: "I'm surprised you even have to ask. Which organization provides and underwrites, or has historically provided and underwritten the majority of continuing medical education programs for US physicians and physician extenders (nurse practitioners and physician assistants) after they complete their medical training?"

Tennyson: "The pharmaceutical industry?"

Worthington: "Correct. And why is that?"

Tennyson: "Well, if you believe the feds and some of the naïve general public that has been misled by those ill-informed and self-righteous dingbats, it's because Big Pharma believes it can manipulate doctors into writing inappropriate prescriptions merely by giving them a pen or an occasional free lunch."

Brand: "And if you ignore that obviously ignorant and insulting sentiment?"

Tennyson: "It's because both organizations need each other. Medicine and Big Pharma are, to use a modern term, the ultimate life partners. Without prescription medications and fancy surgical devices, organized medicine is reduced to the relatively useless role of hand-holding and death-predicting it once held; and without healthcare providers prescribing their products, the pharmaceutical industry is out of business."

Worthington: "Exactly. So how does this play into our tumultuous testosterone tale?"

Brand: "Well, it suggests that doctors and other medical providers will remain relatively naïve about the subject until the pharmaceutical industry starts marketing testosterone products to the medical community. Speaking of which, I've recently been seeing ads for some testosterone creams and gels—including one you use like an underarm deodorant. Shouldn't that get the ball rolling?"

40

Worthington: "One would hope so. *He pauses because he is obviously confused.* I guess I find this subject perplexing."

Tennyson: "How so?"

Worthington: "What's the hottest medical topic in the news today? What's the disease you can't turn on a radio or TV, or open a newspaper or magazine without hearing about?"

Brand: "I don't know…breast cancer?"

Worthington: Alan, how many people died in the US in 2012 from all cancers combined?"

Brand: "No idea…half, three quarters of a million?"

Worthington: "Not bad. My machine here says 575,000. Dr. Tennyson, now to your wheelhouse: How many people died in the US in 2012 from cardiovascular disease?"

Tennyson: *Responds immediately without hesitation.* "That number would be exactly 597, 689 souls, sir."

Worthington: "Are you two suggesting that a condition like low testosterone syndrome, that contributes to the largest killer in what is supposed to be the world's most highly developed nation, namely heart disease, is essentially being ignored.

Brand: "Appears that way, Sam."

Worthington: "How can that be?"

Brand: "As a family physician, Sam, you, of all people, surely know that answer better than any of us. It's because men don't go to the doctor. They don't go because they are raised to be stoic and tough out whatever ails them,

41

whether it's a hangnail, a rattlesnake bite, or a skin cancer that has eaten off half of their arm."

Tennyson: "And that's not the only reason they don't go. Men avoid physicians and hospitals because, while we like to think we're all macho tough guys who fear nothing, we actually do fear four things: God, the IRS, angry women, and doctors. As to the seemingly exaggerated media attention to breast cancer, it's probably because women are better organizers than we are; they are a group that once had no social or political voice, so they worked hard to earn that voice. The extraordinary breast cancer awareness campaign of the past twenty-some years is testimony to this. Men should take a lesson from women. What is needed to increase public knowledge of the relationship between testosterone levels and men's overall health is an aggressive awareness campaign!"

Worthington: "I can just see the placards at the rallies now: 'Hell no, we won't go 'cause our testosterone is low!'"

Brand: *Chuckling.* "Or 'We'd get (it) up ourselves, but we can't!'"

Tennyson: *Smiling, but serious.* "We laugh, but this is obviously no laughing matter. It sounds like men's lives are being maimed by the serious health risks that accompany low testosterone syndrome and ED, and most don't even know anything about the connection to serious medical problems. What they know is that their sex life is affected by ED; what they don't know is that ED is screaming at them to run to the doctor immediately and get checked for heart, circulatory, diabetes, blood pressure, depression, hormone and other possible medical problems. Not only is this condition about which they are unaware, wreaking havoc on their personal and professional life and overall health, this silent, toxic force may also be sending them to an early grave. Talk about killing me softly! I remember more than once hearing my daddy say, 'Not right now, Roly, my sap's a bit low today.' Sounds like my Pops knew more biology than he let on!"

HORMONE BASICS

Before we begin our discussion about the role testosterone plays in men's health, it makes sense to make sure you possess a basic understanding of hormones. Hormones are chemical messages, or physiologic signals, produced by glands. These messages are relayed from the gland that produces them to another organ, gland or body part to effect an action. Restated, hormones are a message from one organ that tells other organs what do. Since testosterone is the hormone of primary interest in this book, let's review an example of the physiologic process that results in the increased levels of testosterone required for an adolescent male to enter puberty:

1) The brain sends a signal to the testes to increase testosterone production.

2) The testes receive the message and increase production of testosterone.

3) Testosterone is released from the testes and enters the bloodstream.

4) These elevated testosterone levels result in the young man experiencing the physical, sexual and emotional changes associated with puberty such as weight gain; bone and muscle growth; development of facial,

armpit, and pubic hair; increased height; emotional lability; increased interest in the opposite sex; wet dreams; increased erections; penis and testicle enlargement; and so on.

5) Upon completion of puberty the body signals the brain that the extremely elevated levels of testosterone required for puberty are no longer needed. The brain then sends a message to the testes to make and release less testosterone.

To make doubly sure you understand the basic concept of hormones, let's review insulin's role in blood sugar regulation and why a deficiency, or imbalance, of this hormone results in the extremely common medical condition known as *diabetes*.

1) The body sends a signal to the *pancreas* (the organ where insulin is made and stored) that the person's blood sugar level is low.

2) The pancreas receives the message and releases insulin into the bloodstream.

3) Insulin is taken up and used by the large number of cells in the body that require insulin to function.

4) The body senses that blood sugar levels are now normal and insulin levels are adequate, so sends a message back to the pancreas that it has received enough insulin.

5) The pancreas reduces the amount of insulin it is releasing.

Another important definition is *hormone balance*.
Hormone balance means that the amount, or blood

level, of a hormone in your body remains at levels needed for you to function properly. Two criteria must be satisfied for hormone balance. First, your measured hormone level (determined by blood or saliva test) must be at or near the recommended levels. Second, you cannot be experiencing the symptoms associated with the hormone being out of balance (too high or low). Restated, your hormones are out of balance, or in a state of *hormone imbalance*, if the hormone or hormones in question <u>are not</u> at or near recommended levels and you <u>are</u> experiencing the symptoms consistent with their being too high or too low.

Let's look at how examples of testosterone balance and testosterone imbalance differ to better illustrate this idea.

<u>Hormone balance</u>: A 49 year-old male businessman named Jack feels fine, but his loving wife saw a commercial touting the benefits of a new testosterone cream on Low T. Upon hearing the potentially devastating health ramifications of what the announcer called *Andropause* (another name for low testosterone syndrome, Low T), his wife demanded Joe undergo evaluation to make sure he was not being silently sucked to an early grave by this dreaded condition. Jack, ever the obedient husband, went to the doctor where he was found to have no symptoms consistent with andropause and his blood tests revealed his total testosterone level to be 800 (250 to 1,100 is normal for the lab where his test was performed), and his free testosterone level was 15.5 (7-25 is the normal range in this same lab). Since Jack's testosterone levels were normal and he had no symptoms of andropause, his testosterone level is balanced; ergo, he is in a state of *testosterone balance.*

<u>Hormone imbalance</u>: Bill, a 54 year-old factory worker, has felt like a tire that has been steadily losing air for the past five years and is getting to the point where he can hardly muster the energy to get up and go to work, let alone work effectively when he's there. He stumbled upon a low testosterone website when searching the term *fatigue* on the Internet. He was shocked to find that he had almost all of the possible symptoms seen in Andropause, so contacted the anti-aging medical practice that sponsored the Internet site. Unlike Jack, his total testosterone level was seriously low at 125 (250 to 1,100 is normal in this lab, also), and his free testosterone level was quite low at 6.6 (Again, 7-25 is the normal range). Unlike Jack, both of Bill's measured testosterone levels <u>were</u> abnormal and he <u>did have</u> many symptoms of Andropause. By definition, because he has symptoms of Andropause and his lab results are those seen in Andropause, he suffers from *testosterone imbalance.*

There's one final thing you need to understand about hormones, wellness and male health before going further into our discussion about testosterone. Hormones are classified based on the way they are produced. These two hormone classifications are (1) synthetic and (2) bioidentical.

The introduction of bioidentical hormones is changing the way today's enlightened healthcare providers approach the treatment of hormone imbalance. What are *bioidentical hormones?* Bioidentical hormones are hormones that are exactly the same as those made by the body. They are considered *natural* because they come from nature (they are made from soy and yams) and are *molecularly identical*—or biologically the same—as the hormones made by our bodies.

In contrast to "natural" bioidentical hormones, *synthetic* (artificial), or non-bioidentical, hormones created in laboratories by large pharmaceutical companies, are not molecularly identical to the hormones our body produces. This distinction is important because the body can distinguish between a scientifically engineered hormone that is close to what it is used to seeing and the Real McCoy. The human body is the most extraordinary, exacting and precise machine ever made and won't fall for this ill-conceived attempt at molecular impersonation, just as you wouldn't be fooled by somebody wearing a disguise who was attempting to trick you into believing they are your spouse or child or parent. Because precise cellular recognition of hormones by *target glands* (the gland or glands the hormone is supposed to affect) is critical to effective hormone action, synthetic (artificial) hormones that masquerade as the hormones the body expects to see, do not yield the same hormonal effects that bioidentical hormones do. Unfortunately, this misrecognition leads to reduced hormone efficacy and possible side effects, some of which can be severe. The testosterone molecule examples below illustrate the molecular differences between bioidentical testosterone and a leading synthetic testosterone.

BIOIDENTICAL VS SYNTHETIC TESTOSTERONE HORMONE

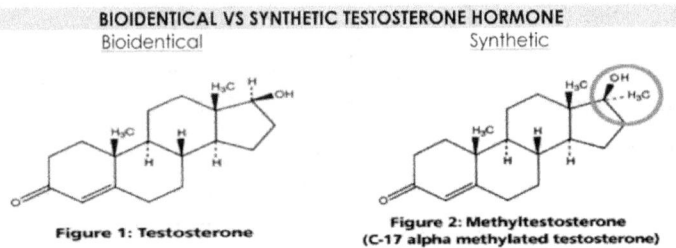

BIOIDENTICAL VS SYNTHETIC TESTOSTERONE HORMONE
Bioidentical   Synthetic

Figure 1: Testosterone

Figure 2: Methyltestosterone
(C-17 alpha methylated testosterone)

Note how the area of the molecule inside the circle in the compound on the <u>right</u> side (synthetic compound) differs from the same area in the upper right hand of the compound on the <u>left</u> side (bioidentical compound). The bioidentical testosterone molecule on the left is exactly the same as the testosterone produced by our bodies; the synthetic molecule on the right is not. This is important because the body's hormone recognition system is so sensitive that one tiny little molecular difference will interfere with the body's ability to recognize the molecule, resulting in poor hormone effect, side effects and disease.

TESTOSTERONE

Testosterone plays critical roles throughout a man's life. Scientists classify this hormone produced by the testes and adrenal glands as an *androgen* (*andro*: male; *ogen:* suffix denoting hormone), because it is the driving biological force behind *masculinization.* Its presence causes the physical and mental changes associated with becoming and being an adult male, such as increased body and facial hair, deepening of voice, bone growth, muscle bulk, development of male genitalia, aggressive and assertive territorial male behavior, libido (sex drive), and sperm production by the testes. It is also essential for maintenance of self-esteem, mental sharpness, memory, concentration, sexual performance, and preventing weight gain, strokes, heart attacks, osteoporosis and diabetes.

Testosterone deficiency, a syndrome that also goes by the names of *Testosterone Deficiency Syndrome, Andropause,* and *Low T,* is a very common and destructive medical condition. It is the male equivalent of menopause, but begins developing earlier than the well-known feminine version of sex hormone balance, with most male sufferers beginning their testosterone decline in their late 20s or early

48

30s. The list of physical signs, symptoms, and medical conditions associated with testosterone deficiency is both lengthy and worrisome as seen in the table on the next page.

LOW TESTOSTERONE SYNDROME		
Fatigue	Increased exercise	Testicular atrophy
Sleep difficulty	recovery time	(shrinking)
Low energy	Body aches	Decreased libido
Decreased self-esteem	Memory problems	Lowered self-confidence
Hair loss	Sexual difficulties	Muscle loss
Irritability	Erectile dysfunction (ED)	Increased risk of:
Depression	Breast pain or	• heart attack
Anxiety	enlargement	• stroke
Moodiness	Weight gain	• blood clots
Infertility	Joint aches and pains	• diabetes

Many people who have difficulty accepting the relatively recently discovered scientific truth that menopause has a masculine counterpart, find it helpful to compare the symptoms of Andropause with those of menopause in females seen in the table below. The parallels between the two conditions are eerie, but this shouldn't surprise us because both are the biological result of declines of the respective sex hormones that differentiate the two genders. Deficiencies of estrogen and progesterone result in Menopause, and deficiency of testosterone results in Andropause.

MENOPAUSAL SYNDROME (MENOPAUSE)		
Fatigue	Increased exercise	Hair loss
Sleep difficulty	recovery time	Painful intercourse
Low energy	Body aches	Decreased libido
Decreased self-esteem	Memory problems	Muscle loss
Lowered self-confidence	Sexual difficulties	Breast shrinkage
Irritability	Vaginal dryness	Increased risk of:
Depression	Breast pain or	• heart attack
Anxiety	enlargement	• stroke
Moodiness	Weight gain	• blood clots
Infertility	Joint aches and pains	• diabetes

DIAGNOSING TESTOSTERONE DEFICIENCY

Diagnosing a hormone imbalance requires that your medical provider know your medical history, elicit your physical and mental symptoms, and perform a physical examination. If these suggest a problem, laboratory testing (saliva/or blood) is used to confirm the suspected condition or conditions. In addition, a *PSA*, or Prostate-specific antigen test, and a digital rectal examination should be performed as screens for presence of prostate cancer. If your PSA number is high, your healthcare provider will likely perform follow-up testing to make sure you do not have prostate cancer. The current medical understanding regarding testosterone replacement and prostate cancer is that prostate cancer is not caused by treating low testosterone syndrome with testosterone replacement therapy, but if you do have prostate cancer, the cancer will likely grow faster if you take supplemental testosterone.

The way testosterone exists in the human body male is unique. *Total testosterone* is the total amount of testosterone present in the body. Laboratories arrive at this lab value (number) by adding the quantities of the two forms in which testosterone exists in the body: (1) *Protein-bound testosterone*, or testosterone molecules that are not biologically available for immediate use because a protein molecule is bound (stuck) to them; and (2) *Free testosterone*, or biologically available testosterone molecules that do not have a protein molecule stuck to them and so are available for immediate use by the body. *Protein binding* is a critical component of many physiological processes—especially as regards hormones—because proper hormone levels and function require adequate body protein levels. Persons suffering from protein deficiency of any cause often develop protein binding problems that interfere with their hormone levels, a situation that often compounds their health woes.

Because *free testosterone* is the amount of testosterone the body can actually use, it's the lab test most healthcare providers rely on most heavily when diagnosing and treating testosterone imbalance.

The Professor Says:

Total Testosterone =
Free testosterone (**usable**) + *Protein Bound testosterone*
(**unusable**)

TREATING TESTOSTERONE DEFICIENCY

Treatment of testosterone deficiency requires a unique three-component strategy in order to be successful. If this treatment strategy isn't followed, not only will testosterone levels not be optimized, serious and potentially permanent side effects may result. Unfortunately, many well-meaning conventional physicians who have begun treating Andropause patients are not aware of the absolute requirement for this treatment strategy and are therefore unknowingly causing their patients problems, some of which may become irreversible. These three components of Andropause treatment are:

1. Testosterone Replacement Therapy: See discussion below

2. Gonadotropin: Gonadotropins are hormones that stimulate growth and activity of the gonads. The gonads in males are the testicles (testes); female gonads are the ovaries. Gonadotropin replacement is required in Andropause treatment because of the body's *Hormonal Negative Feedback System.* Composed of the gonads and the pituitary gland located in the brain, this feedback system is designed to keep the sex hormones in balance. When the pituitary, which has become accustomed to low testosterone levels (testosterone deficiency, Low T), suddenly senses the dramatic rise in testosterone caused by testosterone replacement, it believes that the testicles have miraculously overcome their previous problems and begun making up for lost time by producing high levels of testosterone. The pituitary then signals the testes to reduce testosterone production in order to prevent testosterone excess. This normal physiologic response cannot be allowed to happen for two reasons: the first reason is that negative feedback from the pituitary will result in the testicles producing even less testosterone than before, resulting in a worsening of the hormone deficiency state. That production, therefore, must be maintained at all costs. The second reason is even more important. Testicles receiving signals to reduce testosterone production over a sustained period of

time essentially slip into a dormant state, causing them to atrophy (shrink up to nothing). And eventually become unable to produce testosterone—a condition that can be permanent. If permanent, the man is infertile and will require lifelong testosterone replacement. Most of you have heard the jokes about steroid-abusing bodybuilders ending up as great big boys with little bitty balls. Those jokes exist for a reason, because many of these athletes secured these drugs illegally on the black market and did not know how to use them properly. This misuse resulted in many of them becoming infertile and needing to take testosterone therapy for the rest of their life because they destroyed their body's ability to make testosterone. This sad tale reminds us that testicles must be viewed like any other organ or muscle in the body. Muscles that are exercised regularly stay healthy and grow big and strong; conversely, muscles that are ignored or not exercised regularly wither away and become useless. "Use 'em or lose 'em" is the operative phrase as regards testicles and testosterone production.

The medications (gonadotropins) commonly prescribed to prevent the pituitary from turning off testosterone production are *human chorionic Gonadropin* (hCG), this comes as either an injection drops placed under the tongue (sublingual); and Clomiphene (brand name Clomid®), which comes in pill form.

3. Aromatase Inhibitors: Aromatase inhibitors are used in the treatment of low testosterone syndrome to inhibit the enzyme, *aromatase*. Aromatase is responsible for converting testosterone to estrogen. As crazy as it sounds, giving testosterone to a man

without an aromatase inhibitor will usually increase the levels of the "female" hormone, estrogen. All men make and need some estrogen and certain levels of estrogen are required for hormone balance and normal male functioning, but if estrogen levels become too high it can lead to problems. Failure to take an aromatase inhibitor along with supplemental testosterone worsens testosterone:estrogen ratio imbalance, resulting in weight gain, breast enlargement (*gynecomastia*), and possibly a desire to shop in the Ladies section of department stores.

Aromatase inhibitors commonly prescribed for this purpose include *Tamoxifen* (brand names Nolvadex®, Tamofen®, Tamoxen®, Soltamox®) and *Anastrozole* (Arimidex®).

While many methods exist for treating men suffering from testosterone deficiency, most men choose treatment with either injections or creams, because these two time-tested options are safe, effective, relatively inexpensive, and are products the medical community has the most experience with. However, the past few years has seen a steady rise in testosterone pellet placement, as a means for treating testosterone deficiency.

1. Testosterone Pellets is a quick, safe and simple procedure consisting of numbing a small area over the hip with a small shot, making a shallow 3 millimeter incision, and then inserting a number of pellets into a small hole under the skin through a hollow needle called a *trocar*. After the pellets are placed, the incision is closed with Steri-strips. Restrictions of this procedure are mandates to avoid vigorous physical activity for 24 hours and ice the area intermittently on the day of pellet placement. As

with all medical procedures involving breaking the skin, infection is a possible risk, but occurs only rarely.

2. Testosterone injections are given directly into a muscle. Traditionally, men went to their physician's office to receive this treatment. Fortunately, this treatment option has become much more convenient because men can now give themselves these once-weekly injections at home.

3. Testosterone creams and lotions are available for patients who either want to avoid injections or are unable to receive injections for medical or other reasons. Testosterone creams are used daily and tolerated well, with mild acne at the treatment sites a possible side effect.

4. Sublingual drops are a new addition to treatment options for men suffering from testosterone deficiency. Sublingual means "under the tongue". Available at select compounding pharmacies, this recent technological advance avoids the physiologic issue of testosterone deactivation by the liver that occurs with testosterone taken by mouth. This makes it possible to treat testosterone deficiency by giving drops absorbed into the tissue under the tongue. This unique delivery method allows the hormone to be directly delivered into the bloodstream.

5. Pills and capsules are being used for the treatment of testosterone deficiency by innovative healthcare providers and compounding pharmacies. This cutting edge development is big news in the hormone world, as prior attempts at creating testosterone pills or

capsules failed because the orally-delivered hormone would be deactivated by liver metabolism, as it passed through the digestive tract. Like the sublingual drops described above, these exciting new products avoid the liver metabolism and drug deactivation issue that previously prevented treating testosterone deficiency with pills. These new pills unique formulations delay absorption of testosterone until it has progressed far enough down the digestive tract to avoid liver metabolism, where it is absorbed into the bloodstream and results in balanced blood and tissue testosterone levels.

OTHER HORMONES AND MALE SEXUAL HEALTH

Testosterone is not the only hormone critical to maximizing male sexual health. If thyroid, cortisol, DHEA, progesterone and estrogen levels are out of balance, they can negatively affect testosterone levels and can also cause hormone imbalance syndromes that will negatively impact your health.

Hypothyroidism is a hormone deficiency state resulting from destruction of thyroid hormone by disease or underproduction of thyroid hormone by the thyroid gland. The thyroid is located in the neck and plays numerous important roles in human health, including regulation of metabolism, organ and overall body growth, and ensuring proper function of other hormones.

Possible hypothyroidism symptoms include fatigue, weight gain, depression, anxiety, dry skin, hair loss, thinning hair, erectile dysfunction, constipation, puffy face, mental slowing, joint pains, slow heart rate, and heart failure in severe cases. Laboratory testing used to diagnose hypothyroidism includes a thyroid blood panel consisting of TSH (*thyroid stimulating hormone*), T4 (*thyroxine*) and T3 (*triiodothyronine*). This condition, which is more common in women than men, but affects many men nonetheless, can be potentially devastating. Fortunately, it is readily treated with bioidentical thyroid replacement therapy.

Cortisol deficiency is another hormone imbalance that negatively impacts male health and testosterone status. Cortisol is produced by the adrenal glands, which are small organs located on top of either kidney. Imbalance of this critically important hormone results in poor quality of life and even death in severe cases. The two most common causes of *hypocortisolism* (cortisol deficiency) are a condition named *Addison's disease* that results in underproduction of cortisol by defective adrenal glands and *adrenal fatigue*, a symptom complex caused by chronic stress that results in burnout of the adrenal glands that renders them incapable of providing adequate amounts of cortisol for normal human function. Symptoms of cortisol deficiency include fatigue, sluggishness, weight gain, bone and muscle loss, depression, anxiety, feeling tired but wired, foggy thinking, and irritability. Diagnosis of hypocortisolism used to require extensive testing, but can be accomplished for many patients through a simple combination of blood or saliva testing. Fortunately, most patients respond positively to replacement with oral corticosteroid therapy. Examples of corticosteroids include Prednisone, Dexamethasone, and others.

Deficiency of *dehydroepiandrosterone* (DHEA) is another common hormone imbalance that negatively affects men's health. DHEA is produced by the adrenal glands and is an important *precursor*, or intermediate step, in the production of numerous hormones. DHEA deficiency symptoms include fatigue, decreased sex drive, decreased musculature, depression, anxiety, and hair loss, as well as increased risk for heart disease, stroke and memory difficulty. Most cases of DHEA deficiency are due to decreased age-related production of the hormone by the adrenal glands, and treatment options include compounded bioidentical DHEA or the over-the-counter *7-keto DHEA* supplements.

Finally, imbalances of the hormones most people associate with women—progesterone and estrogen—can also harm male sexual health. What is unique about these hormones as regards optimizing men's overall health and wellness is the need to maintain proper ratios of these hormones with testosterone. Recommended testosterone: estrogen ratios range from 30:1 to 40:1. Understandably, the lower the testosterone level, the lower the testosterone: estrogen ratio becomes. Correction of the ratio requires raising the testosterone component and lowering the estrogen component of the ratio. The two keys to correcting this ratio abnormality are (1) increasing the amount of testosterone in the body and (2) preventing conversion of testosterone to estrogen by prescription of an *aromatase inhibitor* (type of drug that prevents testosterone from being converted to estrogen). As previously stated, the body actually converts testosterone to estrogen, a process requiring the presence of the enzyme aromatase. Examples of aromatase inhibitors commonly prescribed for this purpose include *Tamoxifen* (brand names Nolvadex®, Tamofen®, Tamoxen®, Soltamox®) and *Anastrozole* (brand name Arimidex®).

THE TESTOSTERONE—PROSTATE CANCER QUESTION

Just as the misinformation provided to the public on the findings of the *Women's Health Initiative* study on hormone use in menopausal women, caused a tremendous setback for women's healthcare, rumor-mongering about testosterone replacement therapy being a cause of prostate cancer, has resulted in a great deal of unnecessary anxiety among men. This information has prevented an incalculable number of already treatment-shy men, desperately in need of care for their male sexual health problems, from seeking the safe and effective testosterone replacement therapy that would have likely improved both the quality and length of their lives. Interestingly enough, current shifts in thinking suggest an imbalance of the estrogens (estrogen too high, testosterone too low) in the body may be one of the leading culprits for development of prostate cancer. The truth is that testosterone does not cause prostate cancer; however, men who have prostate cancer should not take supplemental testosterone because it will likely worsen their cancer.

Are you interested in looking better, feeling better, and improving your sex life? Go to **www.totalmale.com** to learn more about ED, premature ejaculation, penis enhancement, low testosterone syndrome, prostate health, other male sexual health issues, increased longevity, and improving your overall quality of life.

You can also learn more about your hormones, including total and free testosterone, by reading our book, My Hormones; A simple guide to better and longer living or by visiting our website, **www.myhormones.com**.

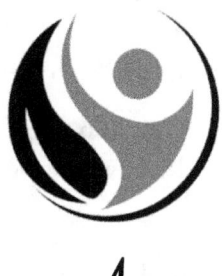

4

Slow down, you move too fast You've got to make the morning last

Man survives earthquakes, experiences the horrors of illness, and all of the tortures of the soul. But the most tormenting tragedy of all time is, and will be, the tragedy of the bedroom.
—Tolstoy

SAVING MENKIND

By A. F. Wells

Act 3

8:00 a.m., Wednesday

Setting: The doctor's lounge again.

Tennyson: "Well, gents, I'd like to call our recently formed men's club of sorts to order by introducing yet another thing of which men do not speak. What say we chat about that oldie, but goodie: premature ejaculation?"

Worthington: "What say we don't, and say we did? Why on God's green earth would you want to wade into those murky waters?"

Brand: "Probably because the heart specialist sitting next to me has been buffing up on his male sexual health issue knowledge since we've created our little club and discovered that not only is premature ejaculation fairly common, affecting around one-third of all men regardless of age, it, like the other conditions we discussed lately, is also quite treatable."

Worthington: "Sure, why not? In for a dime, in for a dollar! We're so far down this bumpy road we might as well push on to the bitter end." *He pauses then chuckles at his joke.* "No pun intended, of course."

Brand: "You are excused, sir, for that lame attempt at humor. Speaking of humor, I'd like to complement all of us for making sure our little soirees haven't turned into a contest to see who can tell the best Viagra® jokes. One of my patients has a handful of new ones every time he comes in. Man, do I hate seeing his name on my schedule!"

Tennyson: "Do you understand, Alan, why men tell those jokes?"

Brand: "Sure, the psychology is quite simple. It's because most of them have one or more of the problems we've been discussing, and making light of the subject helps relieve their fears and anxieties about what they believe to be personal shortcomings that are actually medical problems."

Worthington: "Would one of you amateur psychologists mind beginning a discussion on premature ejaculation?"

Brand: "Happy to oblige, sir. For starters, what's your definition of premature ejaculation?"

Tennyson: "Well, since we all know that if Mama ain't happy, then nobody's happy, I'd have to say it's the man ejaculating before the woman wants him to."

Brand: "Reasonable thinking, Roland, and I would agree with you, but organized medicine has decided that the definition is as simple as 'the man ejaculating before he would like to.'"

Worthington: "Yeah, right. Good luck trying to sell that definition to any of my wife's friends. Any man who has been married as long as I have is quite aware that he who places his own desires—whether they be sexual, recreational, dietary, or any other—before those of his spouse, will soon discover that approaching life in such self-centered fashion quickly leads to his golf clubs and underwear being thrown out the window and his relocation from the blissful marital bed to the unhappy bachelor couch. So fiddlesticks on the governing body's definition; this issue, while it is a male one, is actually about pleasing his significant other. Unfortunately, humans aren't allowed the luxury of being an animal that views mating as something to be done quickly and efficiently in order to minimize exposure to predators; we are one of the few creatures that uses sex and mating not only as a means of reproduction, but also as a way to ensure stability of the mating couple and the family unit."

Brand: "Sam, sounds like you should be leading this discussion, not me. That last bit was worthy of Darwin himself."

Worthington: "It is what it is, my friend. So, moving on…I'll admit that I've never taken the time to learn about diagnosing or treating premature ejaculation because I have never—not once in fifty years of practicing medicine—had a male patient ask about it. I figured that if they weren't asking, they either didn't have it or didn't want to discuss it."

Tennyson: "A rationale I'm confident is espoused by many of our colleagues—and not just as regards this issue. Consider major depression: before the Prozac® revolution, depression and psychiatric medications were taboo subjects. Nowadays, you're not part of the 'it' crowd unless you're taking an antidepressant. Perhaps the same thing will happen with ejaculatory dysfunction."

Brand: "While I suspect you may be a bit 'premature' in your thinking, Roland, the fairly recent paradigm shift regarding erectile dysfunction is encouraging. It still shocks me how quickly that dramatic change to our society's approach to such an incredibly taboo subject occurred. Can you imagine our grandparents discussing ED at one of their bridge parties or company picnics the way people do today?"

Worthington: "Times, they are a changing. You're quite right about that. Since it's now considered okay to discuss ED and low testosterone in social circles, I suspect the logical next step is groups at cocktail parties and church socials engaged in heated conversations about how long a guy can last or publicly discussing his inability to hold back his big moment. If that isn't a sign for the people at the church social that we're approaching the 'end of times,' what is?"

Brand: "Dr. Tennyson, did you learn anything about treatment options for premature ejaculation during your clandestine forays into the subject?"

Tennyson: "As a matter of fact, I did. It looks like the best results are achieved with a combination of counseling (therapy) and medications. It seems the usually undesired sexual side effects of some antidepressants are where the action lies in helping men reduce premature ejaculation issues."

Worthington: "Another win for the antidepressants! Every time I turn around they are being used for something else. Pretty amazing notion to an old codger like me, being that I was trained in that archaic era where depression was considered a defect of the spirit, that it was essentially a lack of gumption. Back then, treatment options consisted of either repeated swift kicks in the pants to aid the morose person into 'getting over it', or packing them off to Trembling Hills for the much needed rest, knitting, crossword puzzles, and social isolation that might help cure their neurosis. As Roland said, in the old days depression was a badge of shame that remained a tightly held family secret; these days it is a red badge of courage worn proudly and loudly."

Brand: "One last question for you two before we adjourn: What are your personal opinions as to why some men have trouble with premature ejaculation and some don't?"

Tennyson: "I'll answer for both of us, because I cheated and looked up the answers to the test before coming today. The answer is that we know orgasm and subsequent ejaculation is a neurophysiological event. In other words, it's a biological reaction resulting from neurochemical actions, which helps explain the value of antidepressants as a treatment, since they act on neurotransmitters (neurochemicals). Most experts believe premature ejaculation ("PE") is a combination of behaviors related to anxieties regarding sex and an inherited predisposition to the condition—that sufferers have a decreased awareness of the biological events heading them towards orgasm and release of ejaculate. As a result, ejaculation sneaks up on them and the show is over only moments after it began."

Brand: "Would an example of your 'behaviors related to sexual anxieties' be a man choosing to go ahead and ejaculate instead of hold back because he feels PE is less embarrassing than experiencing another humiliating episode of ED?"

Tennyson: "Exactly, that's a perfect example! Another one would be a man telling his wife he is too tired for sex, when would actually love to give it a go because he is terrified of disappointing her yet again."

Worthington: "Interesting stuff, guys. But to get back to this newfangled PE definition that says premature ejaculation is when a man finishes before HE wants to, I feel fairly certain that any man who comes home and, as he slips into bed says, to the wife, 'Oh, by the way, honey, I saw my doctor today and he said my problem with being a quick shooter isn't my fault because it's a biological thing I inherited. He said you'll need to get over it because there's nothing to be done!' will likely find himself in dire need of an ice pack and a bottle of aspirin to treat the lump on his head resulting from the frying pan his beloved bride lays upside his head!"

<u>Brand</u>: "Agreed. I'll get you guys some articles that address both the treatment of premature ejaculation and the really hard part, which is getting your patients to talk about it. As we all know, getting a man to go to the doctor is like getting a child to go to the dentist to get a tooth pulled. Men do not want to go, and once there usually say as little as possible in hopes of encouraging rapid escape. Those articles should help you provide your patients the care they and their ladies need."

PREMATURE EJACULATION

Premature ejaculation (PE) occurs when a man experiences orgasm and ejaculates soon after sexual penetration and with minimal penile stimulation. Because there is no uniform time cut-off used to define "premature", some medical governing bodies have created their own definitions. These include the International Society for Sexual Medicine's "Ejaculation which always or nearly always occurs prior to or within about one minute" and the International Classification of Diseases (ICD-10) determining the magic number to be a cut-off of 15 seconds from beginning of intercourse. While no worldwide consensus has been reached, the numbers used in these definitions regarding time spent in sexual intercourse prior to male ejaculation are small, with all suggesting extremely brief episodes of intercourse that leave the woman frustrated and the man humiliated.

Ironically, although premature ejaculation is the least-discussed of the male sexual dysfunctions, it is one of the most prevalent. While exact prevalence rates of PE are difficult to determine, the *Sex in America* surveys performed in 1999 and 2008 by University of Chicago researchers, found that 30% of men between adolescence and age 59 reported having experienced PE at least once during the previous 12 months, whereas only about 10% reported erectile dysfunction (ED).

While ED becomes men's most prevalent sex problem after age 60, premature ejaculation remains a significant concern affecting 28% of men age 65 to 74, and 22% of those between the ages of 75 to 85. Other studies report PE prevalence ranging from 3% to 41% of men over 18, but most studies estimate this condition plagues 20% to 30% of males—reaffirming PE as men's most common sex problem.

There is a common misconception that younger men are more likely to experience premature ejaculation than older men and that its frequency decreases with age. This, however, is not true, as PE rates are nearly identical across all age groups.

Premature ejaculation, then, is when a man ejaculates sooner during sexual intercourse than he or his partner would like. Most men have one or more episodes of PE during their life, and as long as it occurs rarely, should not be deemed cause for concern. However, if you develop a consistent pattern of ejaculating sooner than you and your partner wish—such as before intercourse begins or shortly afterward—it is considered premature ejaculation.

As with erectile dysfunction or low testosterone syndrome (Low T), men with PE should not feel they are alone with their problem. Premature ejaculation is a common sexual complaint, with as many as one-third of men affected. Fortunately, although PE is a condition many men feel embarrassed to discuss, it's not only common, it can be improved with treatment.

Some men who think they have PE actually do not. The average time from beginning of intercourse to ejaculation is generally about five minutes, with typical *ejaculatory latency* (time from entry into the vagina to ejaculation) 4 - 8 minutes. While most men with PE often report emotional and relationship distress (some completely stop pursuing sexual relationships) due to PE-related embarrassment, many find it surprising to learn that women tend to consider PE less of a problem than does their partner. This is not to suggest that PE is not distressful for their female partners, but suggests men tend to overestimate the amount of angst it causes their mate.

TREATING PREMATURE EJACULATION

For most men, PE results from a combination of physical and psychological factors. Because of this, treatment options address both of these problem areas.

Behavioral treatment options include the old stand-by of *thinking about something else* during the act of intercourse. Common mental exercise suggestions for inhibiting the most rapid of premature ejaculators include concentrating on the following list of fabulously non-sexual subjects: your grandmother in slinky undergarments, baseball, Warren Buffett wearing nothing but a G-string, Don Rickles in a tutu, practicing multiplication tables, and anything else you can come up with that might distract any neurochemical in the human body and mind whose purpose is facilitating orgasm and ejaculation. What goes unsaid, unfortunately, is that while engaging in these mental tasks may increase duration of intercourse, it will likely do little to improve the pleasure you receive from sexual activity.

Other behavioral activities some men find helpful are:

1) <u>Masturbating prior to intercourse</u>: This activity is only useful if you are able to quickly achieve another erection capable of completing intercourse, so is unlikely to be helpful if you also suffer from ED.

2) <u>Topical desensitizing creams</u>: Good for her, but not so good for you because the creams, by definition, reduce feeling in the penis.

3) <u>Start-stop technique</u>: Immediately withdrawing the penis from the vagina as soon as you sense the first signals of impending orgasm. Unfortunately, this technique of *coitus interruptus* is associated with the risk of ejaculating soon after the hasty retreat from the confines of the vagina is achieved, a result most couples find even less desirable than PE.

4) <u>Squeeze Technique</u>: This behavioral technique involves removing the penis from the vaginal canal upon sensing impending orgasm and then squeezing the tip of the penis. Squeezing the tip of the penis inhibits the orgasm/ejaculation reflex. Once the impulse to ejaculate is quieted, the penis can be reinserted and intercourse restarted.

5) <u>Quiet Vagina</u> is a final method many couples find helpful. This technique minimizes penis stimulation by requiring the male to lie on his back and the female to straddle him, place his penis in her vagina, and then she remains absolutely still. Designed to help increase the amount of time the male spends inside the vagina before ejaculation, this technique can be combined with one or more of the above behavioral approaches to PE.

If you are like most people, you want a pill to fix your problem, whether the problem be ED, PE, VD, MRSA or any other medical acronym. Happily, numerous premature ejaculation treatment options are available in pill form, and most are antidepressants. Why antidepressants? First, as discussed previously, PE is a neurophysiological (brain-body) event and antidepressants target neurophysiological abnormalities (chemical imbalances). Second, while oral antidepressants are safe and effective options for treating depression, anxiety, and other mental health issues, one possible negative aspect associated with them is their potential to cause sexual side effects that include ED and orgasm problems, that range from delayed orgasm to complete inability to achieve orgasm. These side effects, while problematic for persons taking them solely for mental health reasons, provide an opportunity for PE sufferers. Instead of viewing these drugs' possible effects on orgasm as an "undesired side effect", you should, instead, view these effects as a "desired positive effect" on ED.

While most antidepressants and some other psychiatric drugs tend to cause sexual side effects, the medications most often employed in the treatment of premature ejaculation are *Clomipramine* (Anafranil®), a member of the tricyclic antidepressant class; and some members of the selective serotonin reuptake inhibitor class, also known as the *SSRIs*. Members of the SSRI class used in the treatment of PE include *Paroxetine* (Paxil®), *Sertraline* (Zoloft®), *Fluoxetine* (Prozac®), and *Citalopram* (Celexa®).

Some men, although eager to learn about ways to reduce their problems with ED, are hesitant to take an antidepressant as part of their ED treatment regimen, because of side effect concerns or other fears such as social stigma or worries about addiction. Such concerns are

71

generally unfounded because these drugs are not addictive and are safe if taken as directed. The most common side effects of antidepressants are:

- *Neurasthenia:* a mild sense of not caring or worrying about usual life troubles. Often referred to as the "don't give a damns", this side effect is often considered a desirable treatment bonus by men who experience it.

- weight gain;

- sedation (mild), weakness or dizziness

- nausea

- problems with erection

- *anorgasmia*—complete inability to achieve orgasm

There are no hard and fast rules regarding antidepressant dosing treatment regimens in ED. Determining what pill to take, how much and how often to take it are up to you and your healthcare provider. There is little to suggest that daily dosing works better than choosing a "day of the event only" strategy. What works for you is what you should do. Some men find they do better if they take the medication on a daily basis, while others find they do just as well taking it only on days they plan to engage in sexual intercourse. Three things to keep in mind when selecting a treatment regimen: (1) You are more likely to experience side effects if you take the antidepressant on an everyday basis than if you only take it occasionally. These effects usually improve or completely resolve with time or dose reduction and completely leave when you quit using them; (2) the flip side of this equation is that many men who do not think they are depressed or have problems with anxiety, often experience unexpected mental improvement when taking an antidepressant for ED (in medicine this is called unmasking unsuspected depression); (3) choosing to only take your pill on days you "plan" to have intercourse creates the potential for having to pass up an opportunity when an "unexpected opportunity" occurs.

Other less frequently used treatment options include Viagra® and SS-Cream®. The scientific explanation for Viagra®'s positive effect on premature ejaculation is not understood, but suspicions run high it may be due to the medicine's effect on reducing anxieties related to erectile dysfunction. *SS-Cream®* is an herbal desensitizing cream applied to the tip of the penis. Containing nine different herbs, SS-Cream® provides an option for men seeking a "natural" treatment for their PE but, as with all desensitizing creams, it reduces the pleasurable aspect of the activity.

Are you interested in looking better, feeling better, and improving your sex life? Go to **www.totalmale.com** to learn more about ED, premature ejaculation, low testosterone syndrome, penis enhancement, prostate health, other male sexual health issues, increased longevity, and improving your overall quality of life.

To learn more about your hormones, read our book, My Hormones; A simple guide to better and longer living or visit our website, **www.myhormones.com**.

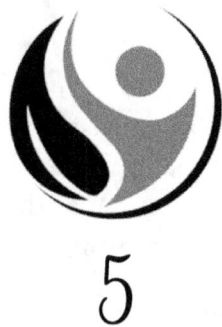

5

Prostate: friend or foe?

It is a great mystery that though the human heart longs for Truth, in which alone it finds liberation and delight, the first reaction of human beings to Truth is one of hostility and fear!
—Anthony de Mello

———————

SAVING MENKIND

By A. F. Wells

Act 4

6:00 p.m., Thursday

Setting: The doctor's lounge. It is empty due to the late hour, so the group is gathered at the main dining table.

Brand: "Thanks, all, for agreeing to meet on such short notice. My last case today got me thinking that one piece of the men's sexual health pie we've neglected to discuss is that most mysterious and widely misunderstood of male organs—the prostate."

Tennyson: "Boy, you can say that again. There are more urban myths floating around about the prostate than Jimmy Hoffa's disappearance! Why do you think that is? What's with the public's problem regarding the prostate?"

Brand: "I have a strong suspicion that it may start with that infamous socially irregular and physically uncomfortable ten-second period involving the doctor's finger and examination of the organ in question."

Tennyson: "What is with the bizarre aura of confusion and mystery surrounding the prostate? How does a tiny gland only the size of a large walnut—a gland nobody ever sees except urologists—evoke such a powerful emotional response?"

Worthington: "Roland, I'm not sure 'powerful response' is the right term. I think the public's odd method of 'handing the prostate issue', for lack of better terms, boils down to a combination of two things: First and foremost being the ancient maxim that people—men especially—tend to fear what they don't understand, which leads into a second truism that men don't want to know anything unsettling as regards their health. What they prefer—and they prefer it even if they know choosing to remain ignorant about the health issue at hand may kill them—is to blindly plod on and not experience interruptions in their daily routine of reading the morning paper, going to and returning from their job, sitting down to dinner with their wife and family, watching a little television in the evening, and then falling asleep fat and relatively happy in their comfortable bed next to their once-blushing bride. And all so they can wake up and do it again the next day."

Brand: "And the second thing?"

Worthington: "It's obvious, don't you think? That fabled institution they have been taught to trust, Organized Medicine, has let them down. Over the past thirty years we failed to provide accurate and consistent messages regarding the prostate. And what makes this failure doubly devastating is that the homely, ugly prostate is like the kid at school who doesn't fit in with any of the other groups. Even though he's part of the male reproductive system, he's not sexy or naughty enough to be included with those flashy sex organs like the vagina, penis, breasts, clitoris, et cetera; and not un-sexy, or basic, enough to run with the kidneys, intestine, lungs, heart, pancreas, and thyroid. Poor old prostate is forced to stand outside the window and press his nose to the cold glass and watch the other kids play the game inside. I kind of feel sorry for him."

Tennyson: "Sam, do try and remember this is a gland we're discussing, not an abandoned puppy."

Brand: "Sam, we've already agreed that one of the major stumbling blocks in helping men conquer their sexual health issues is overcoming their reticence to face them. I'm interested in learning more about this 'failure to communicate' idea of yours as regards the prostate. Would you mind enlightening us?"

Worthington: "Happy to. However, before I answer your question I'd like one of you to tell me what you believe to be the most important role a physician plays in their patients' lives."

Tennyson: "Well…since none of us is Jesus or Mohammed or Buddha, which means we can't cure everything that walks through the door, 'curing disease' can't be the correct answer. That leaves educating the public about health, wellness, and disease. The effective physician/medical provider must be able to communicate and convert complicated scientific ideas into simple, easy-to-understand information for his patients. If he or she can't do that, the majority of their patients will stumble through life, completely bewildered by their bodies, how to take care of them, and what to do if something goes wrong."

Worthington: "Quite the noble and extremely accurate sentiment, Dr. Tennyson. However, to get back to the second reason for the confusion surrounding the prostate, if Organized Medicine was the coach of the Prostate Football Team, it would have been fired long ago for poor performance. Let's consider the list of fumbles it has made during its bumbling efforts to educate the public about the prostate gland and treating prostate conditions: For starters, how many men have been rendered impotent as a result of surgeries for prostate cancer and prostate enlargement? If you want people to develop a negative attitude about an organ, make sure the treatments for this organ—a thing they can't see, feel, or touch—cause them to lose one of the most important things in their life. Two, the way medicine has handled the PSA test is a crime. First we hail it as the holy grail of prostate disease, the simple blood test that instantly tells us whether or not a man has prostate cancer, and then, to raise our level of enthusiasm even further, proclaim that this glorious test may eliminate the need for the rectal exam—the simple and effective test that men say they would rather die than undergo because it violates one of the most sacred mores of the male tribe. The PSA not only created the possibility of eliminating the universally-feared test (DRE) that prevented men from even considering going to a physician's office once they reached the age of 40 (The Prostate Exam Zone), it also carried with

78

it the hope that men and their spouses could feel more secure about an issue that caused so much anxiety and grief. And then, to provide the *coup de gras* to this hate-the-prostate formula, a few years later we—the group entrusted with providing them accurate information they can trust—slap society in the face when we tell them, 'Sorry, folks. Remember all that fabulousness about the PSA being the 'be all, end all test' for prostate issues? It appears that story was just a fairy tale based on bad information and we might have overstated our claims about it.'

"Not only have we lost confidence in using the PSA test to screen for prostate cancer or monitor prostate cancer, we're kind of at the point where most physicians no longer know what to do with it whatsoever. And the final straw is this nonsense about testosterone causing prostate cancer. I mean, Jiminy Cricket!—during the past fifteen to twenty years we've been on the cusp of a scientific revolution that's changing the way we view health and wellness (I'm referring to the role of hormone balance as a critical component of good health here)—and we blunder once again and imply men shouldn't treat the hormone imbalance wreaking havoc on many of their lives and resulting in their early demise. Why not? Because of an outdated and unproven theory that treating them for low testosterone syndrome will likely kill them, because we're pretty sure it causes prostate cancer. And, as per usual, it looks like we must once again reverse ourselves and inform them we screwed up again: testosterone appears to have been unjustly accused, and the real hormonal culprit in prostate cancer causation may actually be testosterone being too <u>low</u>—specifically that having a low testosterone: estrogen ratio is where the real risk lies."

<u>Brand</u>: "Don't you think that's a bit harsh, Roland?"

Tennyson: "With all due respect, sir, I think it's worse than that. Guess which researchers have done the lion's share of the work identifying the misinformation regarding testosterone as a cause of prostate cancer?"

Worthington: "The pharmaceutical companies selling testosterone creams?"

Tennyson: "Good guess, but wrong. Much of the new information has resulted from efforts by a combination of conventional docs who chose to risk persecution from medical boards and other governing organizations by thinking outside the 'mainstream medicine' box, along with alternative health providers our elitist group has so roundly dismissed lo all these years. That's right—we're talking about the groups our mainstream medical educational process taught us are charlatans and healthcare imposters. It appears these people we've long considered overly open-minded, strange, odd, and a few other unflattering terms had to rescue us from ourselves on this one. Nice to see them get a feather for their cap. It's long overdue."

Brand: "So what do we do?"

Tennyson: "Simple. We add demystifying the prostate and providing safer, more effective treatments for prostate conditions to our male sexual health to-do list, a list that already includes erectile dysfunction, low testosterone syndrome, and premature ejaculation."

Worthington: "That's a list that should keep us busy for a long time. Actually, this old dog's been looking for a new trick to learn. I'm looking forward to this new adventure. It's high time that men's sexual health issues were placed front and center. It's clear that most men's approach of benign neglect isn't working for them, so let's help correct the situation. This situation needs a hero, and the definition of a hero is someone who does what needs to be done when it needs to be done, regardless of consequences. So mount up men, today we ride! You guys with me?"

Tennyson and Brand: *Jointly.* "Absolutely, Doctor W, let's go spread the word!"

THE PROSTATE

The *prostate* is a rubbery organ located below the bladder that provides much of the fluid known as *semen,* the liquid substance that serves as the transport medium and nutrition for sperm. *Sperm* is produced in the testicles, and is stored and matures in the *epididymis,* which is a single, tightly coiled tube which lies on top of the testicles and connects the testicles to the *vas deferens.* The vas deferens (the organ surgeons interrupt [cut or burn] during a *vasectomy* to make a man infertile) are paired tubes that transfer sperm to the *seminal vesicles* in preparation for ejaculation. The seminal vesicles are located behind and near the bottom of the *urinary bladder.* The seminal vesicles also contribute fluid to semen, which collects the remainder of the seminal fluid (contributed by the prostate) during its passage through the *urethra* during ejaculation.

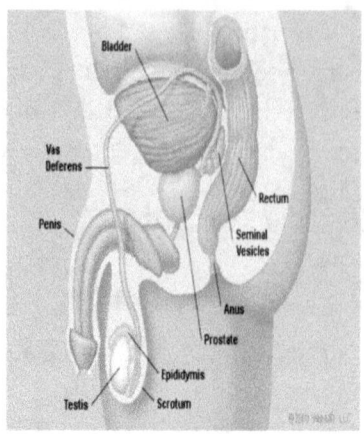

There it is, then. Reproduction is the only reason men have a prostate. The only purpose of the well-hidden gland responsible for a long list of miseries, including urinary difficulties associated with *benign prostate hypertrophy* (*BPH* or non-cancerous prostate enlargement); pain, fever, fatigue, malaise associated with the extremely difficult-to-treat condition known as *chronic prostatitis* (combination of infection and inflammation of the prostate); erectile dysfunction and other male sexual health issues resulting from surgeries and other medical procedures on the gland; the pain, anxiety, disability and death associated with prostate cancer, is performing one of the final steps in the process of producing healthy sperm for making babies.

Other than perpetuation of the species, the prostate is essentially a useless body part, an irritating relative you should kick out of your life the second it's no longer needed. Makes you wonder why doctors don't handle the prostate issue the way they do the uterus in women: surgically remove it to prevent the above problems? The answer, unfortunately, is that prostate surgeries can leave men incontinent and/or impotent—severe conditions that negatively affect quality of life which most men would be unwilling to risk, in order to prevent problems that may never occur.

Three disease processes commonly affect the prostate and men's sexual health. *Benign prostatic hyperplasia*, better known by the acronym, *BPH*, is non-cancerous enlargement of the prostate gland. If the prostate becomes large enough, it compresses the urethra and causes urinary difficulties because the urethra passes through the center of the prostate. An analogy that helps many men understand BPH's problematic effects on urine flow—effects including difficulty starting urination, feeling as if you can't completely empty your bladder, dribbling after urination, increased number of urinary tract infections, having to get up multiple times per night to urinate, and the possibility of being completely unable to urinate—is to picture a straw that passes through an apple. If the apple grows, it grows in all directions, including inward. This inward growth compresses, or pushes on the straw, effectively shrinking the straw's diameter (tube size), which reduces ability of fluid to pass through the straw.

While the infamous and somewhat confusing PSA (prostate specific antigen) test is sometimes elevated in men with BPH, the digital rectal exam is the best way to diagnose this condition. Happily, men with BPH are not at increased risk for developing prostate cancer.

Historically, most cases of BPH that became severe enough to cause significant symptoms were treated surgically with a medical procedure called *trans-urethral resection of the prostate* (TURP). In a TURP, a lighted tube is inserted into the urethra through the tip of the penis. The tip of this tube contains special cutting instruments that allow the surgeon to remove the excess prostate tissue compressing the urethra, thus restoring the diameter of the urethra and improving urinary flow. Although still employed in severe cases of BPH, its use is declining in favor of less-hazardous laser treatments. Currently, most men with BPH are initially treated with two groups of medications known as *alpha-blockers* and *5-alpha reductase inhibitors.* These medications can be given individually or in combination. This decision is based on severity of BPH size and symptoms.

Alpha-blockers, medications whose real scientific drug classification is the complicated phrase ⊠*1-adrenergic receptor antagonists,* reduce BPH symptoms and improve urine flow by relaxing the smooth muscle within the prostate and neck of the bladder. Examples of alpha-blockers, the first two of which are also used in the treatment of high blood pressure, include *Doxazosin* (Cardura®), *Terazosin* (Hytrin®), *Tamsulosin* (Flomax®), and *Silodosin* (Rapaflow®). The most common possible side effect concern with these drugs is dizziness or fainting due to their effects on blood pressure. This can usually be avoided by starting with low doses of the medicine and taking it at bedtime.

5-alpha reductase inhibitors improve BPH symptoms by reducing levels of *dehydrotestosterone* (DHT), a hormone that promotes enlargement of the prostate. The two members of this drug class used in the treatment of BPH are *Finasteride* (Proscar®), also used in the treatment of male pattern baldness under the brand name Propecia®; and *Dutasteride* (Avodart®). Possible side effects of members of this class, including ED, ejaculatory disturbances and decreased libido, result from their effects on testosterone.

Chronic prostatitis plays an important role in men's sexual health, due to the large numbers of men affected, its symptoms, and difficulty both treating and eliminating this irritating and potentially debilitating condition. Chronic prostatitis can be caused by infection, inflammation, or a combination of the two, and its possible symptoms include fatigue, general malaise, pelvic pain, painful urination, penile discharge, ejaculatory disturbances, and flu-like symptoms such as fever, chills, dizziness, headache, and muscle aches.

Because the medical community remains unsure about how to best treat prostatitis, many healthcare providers treat sufferers with a combination of a prolonged course of antibiotics, that concentrates well in the urinary tract and prostate, along with an anti-inflammatory drug such as Naproxen, Ibuprofen, or aspirin. Unfortunately, disease recurrence (relapse) is common, and medical researchers remain diligent in their efforts to solve the riddle of this frustrating and vexing condition that plagues men worldwide.

Prostate cancer is the most common type of cancer in US men. Nearly 300,000 US men are diagnosed annually with prostate cancer, but only one-tenth of this number die from the disease each year. The majority of prostate cancers are diagnosed in men age 65 and older, and most men diagnosed with prostate cancer do not die from the disease. Autopsy studies reveal that 7 in 9 men in their eighties have prostate cancer, a figure that rises to essentially 100% in centurion males. Most of these men never knew they had these cancers, and most died from other causes. Many of these cancers occurring in elderly men grow slowly and are relatively harmless, thus the reassuring phrase cancer physicians often tell these men: "Sir, if you leave it alone, you'll die with prostate cancer, but not from it. If you choose to treat it, you may die from the cancer treatment before whatever it was that was supposed to kill you does you in!"

Unfortunately, the more rapidly growing and thus more lethal versions of the disease, tend to occur in younger men, but are rare in men under 40. As with most cancers, your risk increases if your close relatives have or had it (your prostate cancer risk doubles if your brother or father had the disease). The death toll remains unacceptably high, with prostate cancer running second to lung cancer as the leading causes of cancer death among American men.

Lifetime Probability of a US Male Developing Cancer	
Site	Risk
Prostate	1 in 6
Lung/Bronchus	1 in 13
Colon/Rectum	1 in 19
Bladder	1 in 26
Melanoma	1 in 36
Non-Hodgkin Lymphoma	1 in 43
Kidney	1 in 51
Leukemia	1 in 64
Oral Cavity	1 in 69
Stomach	1 in 91

Until recently, the PSA test was included in annual physical examinations of men 50 years of age and older. However, this recommendation was recently changed because many years of study demonstrate this test may do more harm than good. Unfortunately, large numbers of men with high PSA values ended up going through the unnecessary anxiety, discomfort and possible physical injuries that may result from prostate cancer evaluation, including ED and urinary incontinence, only to discover that they did not have the disease. Disappointingly, this test that healthcare providers initially celebrated for its promise of providing a simple screening solution for early prostate cancer identification, was eventually found to provide results that confused examiners and caused unnecessary stress for patients. Currently, decision-making regarding prostate cancer screening now involves weighing potential risks and benefits of screening. What remains unchanged is the global common sense recommendation that all men participate in a healthy lifestyle that includes regular exercise, a well-balanced diet, plenty of rest, and minimizing stress.

Symptoms, or early warning signs, of prostate cancer may include the urinary difficulties also seen with BPH including trouble starting, stopping, or completing urination, weak or interrupted urine flow, erectile dysfunction, and pelvic or abdominal pain or pressure.

Two tests are used to screen for prostate cancer. Test #1 is the well-known and much-feared digital rectal examination (DRE), the test used by healthcare providers for identifying potentially cancerous lumps on the prostate. In the DRE the physician inserts a lubricated, gloved finger into the rectum and gently palpates the prostate which abuts the rectum. Interestingly enough, most men find the anxiety associated with thinking about the exam much worse than the actual exam itself. Common post-exam reports from patients tend to run along the lines of, "While I wouldn't want to do that every day, it really wasn't that bad. It was just a few seconds of a very strange and slightly uncomfortable pressure that made me want to urinate." Test #2 is the PSA. Again, no longer recommended as a screening test by itself, this test can provide value if the examiner finds a potentially worrisome area on the prostate during the DRE. The PSA detects levels of a protein called prostate-specific antigen and, in general, the higher a patient's PSA level, the greater the likelihood cancer is present. Should the combination of these tests suggest the possibility of prostate cancer, the next step is biopsy of the gland. While biopsy provides no ironclad guarantee, it does provide the best opportunity for knowing whether or not an area of concern is cancerous.

Are you interested in looking better, feeling better, and improving your sex life? Go to **www.totalmale.com** to learn more about ED, premature ejaculation, low testosterone syndrome, penile enhancement, prostate health, other male sexual health issues, increased longevity, and improving your overall quality of life.

To learn more about your hormones, read our book, My Hormones; A simple guide to better and longer living or visit our website, **www.myhormones.com**.

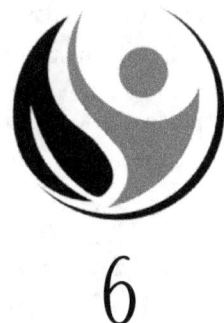

6

Penis Enhancement: Fact or Fiction?

Part of the reason that men seem so much less loving than women is that men's behavior is measured with a feminine ruler.
—Francesca M. Cancian

SAVING MENKIND

By A. F. Wells

<u>Epilogue</u>

6:00 p.m., Thursday

Setting: A cool late summer evening. Dr. Samuel Worthington and his wife, Margaret, have just finished dinner and are relaxing on the front porch in their rocking chairs with a cup of tea.

Samuel: "Marge, I'd like your permission to ask a question that may come off sounding both strange and crude."

Margaret: "What's so special about tonight, Dr. Worthington? If memory serves, you've been a bit strange and crude for about fifty years."

Samuel: *He smiles appreciatively at his bride of almost fifty years.* "Do women discuss penis size? And if they do, what do they say?"

Margaret: "You're right. That is an odd question. What's the deal, Sam, are we developing self-esteem issues? It's a little late in the game for you to be worrying about such things—especially things you can't control."

Samuel: "Therein lies the rub, dearest, because that statement may no longer be true. Please answer my question. I've got a good reason for asking."

Margaret: "First, Sam, there is a small list of things that respectable women do not share with their husband, and the question you just asked would be on that list. Girls must have some secrets, you know! Second, why in blazes would you want to know such a thing?"

Samuel: "Because a patient of mine recently asked my thoughts on whether he should go to one of those new male sexual health clinics to undergo 'male enhancement'."

Margaret: "'Male enhancement'—what's that? Sounds like some kind of right wing extremist boot camp where you learn to be more of a man!"

Samuel: "The answer is that it's a simple in-office procedure where a physician gives a patient a couple of small shots into their penis that increases the size of their penis."

Margaret: "Why in the world would someone do that?"

Samuel: "I suspect for the same reason that women get breast lifts and breast implants—because they aren't satisfied with what they have and aren't interested in allowing nature to take its course, because they know what that looks like."

Margaret: "Yes, but—but…what about things like pain and infection and scarring? Aren't their risks associated with that of medical procedure?"

Samuel: "Good question, dear. My mother told me I was marrying a smart one! Yes, those things and more can occur with any medical procedure. What my research on the issue tells me is that the procedure is quite safe and that pain concerns are relatively minimal."

Margaret: "That's good to hear. But the more important question is, 'Does it work?'"

Samuel: "Based on what I read and a couple of calls I made, I would say the answer is 'Most of the time', but not in a freaky, disturbing kind of way."

Margaret: "Meaning what, exactly?"

Samuel: "Hmmm…how to word such a thing to a classy woman who earlier reminded me that she doesn't tolerate words or subjects usually found in the gutter…?"

Margaret: "Come on—out with it, you old goat! I've been married to family doctor for half a century; I imagine I can handle hearing some silly words like 'penis' and 'longer' and 'wider' and 'harder' uttered in the same sentence."

Samuel: "Yes, ma'am. It looks like most get modest improvement in length and width."

Margaret: "Define 'modest'."

Samuel: "Up to an inch in both dimensions, more or less."

Margaret: *Fans herself in Scarlett O'Hara imitation.* "Oh my, Mr. Worthington, you cause a lady to blush! I may have to repair to the salon to repose. Up to an inch in length and girth? I am impressed!"

Samuel: "Are you serious?"

Margaret: "If you are asking me as a woman whether I like the idea of a man being able to improve his situation, my answer is that life is a game of inches, and every inch counts!"

———————

Many questions plague humanity: Is there a God, Why are we here, Chicken or egg, Yankees or Redsox, and that two-part oldie, but goodie:

(1) Does size matter?
(2) Can anything be done about it?"

The answer to the last question is a resounding "Yes!" Fortunately for men interested in male enhancement, modern medicine now has a solution that helps many achieve their goal of penile enlargement.

For those of you who just muttered, "Yeah, right, Doc! Up to now the book's been great, but you just lost me. I've seen the endless list of ludicrous and salacious penis enlargement ads in magazines and newspapers, and on the internet touting everything from secret sauces to bags of magic beans, as the one miracle method that guarantees a significant and permanent increase in the size of a gentleman's most prized possession. There's no way any of those things work!"

And if you said that, you'd be correct because there are only two guaranteed results from the bizarre collection of penis-enlargement potions, elixirs, pills, powders, devices, exercises, therapies and other remedies to which you allude: the first is that the company selling them will make money; the second is that you're going to be disappointed. Unfortunately, a third possibility is that you might get hurt! It's a long-held business truth that wherever there are people expressing a desire for a product, enterprising gangs of charlatans and hucksters will soon fill that need with an amazing array of useless and potentially dangerous products designed to fleece these unsuspecting victims. Be warned, if you are a man interested in improving your sex life and self-image through penile enlargement, you will not find a credible solution with these products. Happily, however, there are safe, simple, and proven (FDA approved) medical solutions that can help increase penis size.

Prior to considering medical penile enlargement, you should know some basic truths about penis size. A common fear among men is that their penis looks too small and/or isn't large enough to satisfy their partner during sex. If you are one of these men, the following information may help reduce your anxieties about the magnitude of your manhood.

1. Average flaccid (non-erect) penis size is between 3 and 5 inches (8-13 centimeters).

2. Average erect penis size is between 5 and 7 inches (13-18 centimeters).

3. The medical term for a small penis is *micropenis.* In order to be classified as a micropenis, the penis must measure less than 3 inches (7 centimeters) when flaccid.

PENILE ENLARGEMENT: THE LIES

It's critical you understand that nearly all penis enlargement methods are ineffective and while the net result of trying most of them will only be frustration, accompanied by wasted time and money, some can cause injury or scarring that can permanently injure your penis and hinder your ability to perform sexually. If the product you are considering contains the disclaimer, "These statements have not been evaluated by the Food and Drug Administration (FDA)," what that means is that the product you are getting ready to use on your penis has not undergone rigorous testing regarding safety or effectiveness. Would you use a healthcare product on your child or spouse if it contained such a warning? Absolutely not! Considering that the male penis is an extremely important and fragile body part and that injuries to it could be permanent, it stands to reason that if you wouldn't expose your loved ones to a product containing such a disclaimer, it makes absolutely no sense for you to try one of these products because: (1) It has not been proven to work, so it's very unlikely that it will; and (2) there is a real chance you could get hurt.

Below are some examples of these types of products:

Many **lotions and pills** claim to be effective treatments for penile enlargement. These products contain a wide range of ingredients including hormones, minerals, vitamins and herbs, among others. None of these products have been scientifically proven to work because they have not received FDA approval for this condition.

While **vacuum pumps** are an effective treatment for many suffering from erectile dysfunction, they have not been proven to result in permanent penis enlargement. Using a pump can create the momentary illusion of an enlarged penis, but once the pump-induced enlargement resulting from the trapped blood-induced erection resolves, the penis returns to its previous size. This is an example of a potentially dangerous method for penile enlargement because overuse of a vacuum pump can injure elastic tissues in the penis and result in decreased erection firmness.

An example of an exercise touted as being effective for penile enlargement is *Jelqing*. The Jelqing exercise requires that you use a hand-over- hand motion to push blood from the base to the head of your penis. While this unproven method doesn't sound dangerous, it can cause permanent penis scarring, pain and disfigurement so should not be attempted.

Penis stretching is another example of a penis enlargement method to be avoided. While a couple of small scientific studies suggest it can result in up to a 1-inch penis length increase, this method consisting of attaching a stretcher or extender device to the penis is supposed to work by exerting traction on the penis, causing it to become permanently stretch out and thus "lengthened". Thoughts of such a device evoke macabre visions of medieval dungeons, hooded hangmen and the rack. It's no wonder that permanent injuries can result from this treatment method.

For most men, sexual health problems tend to increase as they age. Both physical and mental factors related to aging can have a significant impact on sexual performance. Unfortunately, going back in time is not an option because we have not invented the Time Machine yet. However, there is a safe and relatively effect solution for men seeking penis enlargement and improved sexual function, including ED (see Chapter 2). The **Priapus Shot** ™ is the method of injecting the penis with a substance created from your blood known as Platelet Rich Fibrin Matrix (PRFM). PRFM is created via an exciting new medical technology called *Platelet Rich Plasma* (PRP) being used to help "heal" numerous conditions as wide-ranging as joint replacement, crush injuries of the face, and penile enhancement. One of the unique advances of using this technology to treat penis size and sexual function concerns is that it can rejuvenate and regenerate penile tissue.

PRP's mechanism of action is fascinating and, as previously stated has created an aura of excitement among today's forward-thinking healthcare professionals because of its possibilities for helping a wide range of patients. Such possibilities include spinal cord regeneration that could help paralyzed patients walk or use their arms again; joints that can be healed by a PRP injection instead of painful and debilitating joint replacement; improved hearing and vision among patients with ear and eye damage—who knows where it might lead? Platelets are components of blood critical to the blood-clotting process. They and other components in human blood migrate immediately to a site of injury where they release a variety of factors that respond to tissue injury which initiate and promote healing. By concentrating platelets at the site of injury (PRP), healthcare providers have the potential to enhance the body's natural capacity for healing.

PRP contains growth factors which stimulate the body to repair and restore tissues using its own natural processes. This injection enables penile rejuvenation by promoting increased blood flow to the penis, which ultimately strengthens the erection and enhances appearance. As with all medical procedures, this injection is not guaranteed to help all men who undergo it and has inclusion and inclusion criteria that may result in some men not being able to receive it. Since the patient's own blood is used in this procedure, PRP alleviates the risk of allergic reaction or sensitivity. Other than the usual possible risks associated with any procedure, including pain, swelling, and infection there are no significant risks of using PRP in this way.

The Priapus Shot™—How It Works

- Local anesthetic cream is applied to the injection sites.

- PRP is injected at those precise locations. These treatments rejuvenate the "orgasm system" by stimulating stem cells found in the tissue. New blood vessels and sensory cells are formed and go to work to increase function and improve sensitivity.

- The entire procedure takes less than 15 minutes and requires no downtime.

- Results are typically seen within a week, with many patients experiencing improvements such as increased sensitivity, heightened arousal and improved function within three weeks.

- Many men report increases in firmness of erection, penile length and girth, improved blood flow and circulation, as well as better sexual sensation, pleasure and stamina.

• Men who struggle with sexual dysfunction resulting from prostate enlargement, prostate cancer, surgery, drug side effects or diabetes, may experience nerve regeneration and improved sexual function.

Another option for achieving penile enlargement is surgery. The need for penis-enlargement surgery is rare, with surgery typically reserved for men whose penis doesn't function normally due to birth defect or injury. Penis enlargement surgery for purely cosmetic reasons is considered controversial and because it is more invasive than the injection method describe above, is accompanied by greater risks. A few different surgical techniques are used to lengthen a penis.

1. The most widely used penis-lengthening surgical procedure involves severing the suspensory ligament that attaches the penis to the pubic bone and moving skin from the abdomen to the penile shaft. When this ligament is cut, the penis appears longer because more of it hangs down. However, cutting the suspensory ligament can cause an erect penis to become unstable.

2. Severing the suspensory ligament is sometimes combined with other procedures, such as removing excess fat over the pubic bone.

3. A procedure to make the penis thicker involves taking fat from a fleshy part of the body and injecting it into the shaft of the penis. The results are often disappointing because the injected fat is usually reabsorbed by the body which erases some or all of

the previous "thickening" and can lead to curvature or asymmetry of the penis.

4. Another technique for increasing width is grafting tissue onto the shaft of the penis.

Again, careful consideration is required before undertaking any these potentially harmful procedures.

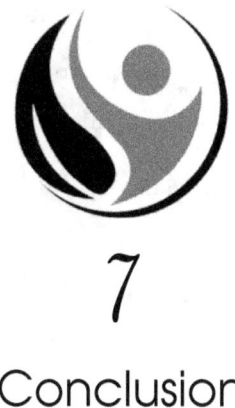

7

Conclusion

Keeping your body healthy is an expression of gratitude to the whole cosmos—the trees, the clouds, everything.
—Thich Nhat Hanh

I t is the sincere hope of the authors that this book helps you better understand male sexual health issues, become aware that safe and effective treatments exist for them, and why addressing any concerns you may have should not only help improve your quality of life and your relationship with your mate—it may also save your life! ***Total Male: Save Your Life by Taking Charge of Your Sexual Health*** is the first in a series of books designed to help men map out a successful approach to health and wellness, with special emphasis on male sexual health issues.

We wish you well on your new adventure, and welcome your comments or questions at our website: **www.totalmale.com**

Sincerely,
Mark Weis, MD and **Douglas Ginter**

Look for our new medical center in San Jose, California

Total Male Medical Center 5595 Winfield Blvd Suite 110 San Jose, California 95123

844-Total-Male or 408-226-2099

info@totalmale.com
www.totalmale.com

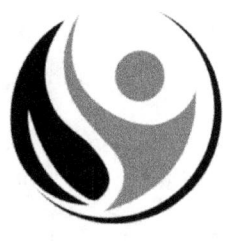

References

AUA guideline on the management of erectile dysfunction: Diagnosis and treatment recommendation. American Urological Association. http://www.auanet.org/content/guidelines-and-quality-care/clinical-guidelines/main-reports/edmgmt/chapter1.pdf. Accessed May 11, 2011.

Coleman, Eli. Erectile Dysfunction: A Review of Current Treatments. *The Canadian Journal of Human Sexuality*, Vol. 7, No. 3.

Heidelbaugh JJ. "Management of erectile dysfunction." *Am Fam Physician*. 2010; 81:305-312.

Jones, J Stephen. *Overcoming Impotence: A Leading Urologist Tells You Everything You Need to Know.* Amherst, NY: Prometheus Books. 2003.

Lee, John R and Hopkins, Virginia. *Dr. John Lee's Hormone Balance Made Simple.* New York, NY: Grand Hatchette Publishing, 2006.

Nikoobakht M, Shahnazari A, Rezaeidanesh M, Mehrsai A, Pourmand G. *Effect of Penile-Extender Device in Increase*

Penile Size in Men with Shortened Penis: Preliminary Results. J of Sex Med; Nov 2011: 8(11):3188-3192.

Siroky MB, Azadzoi KM. *Vasculogenic erectile dysfunction: newer therapeutic strategies.* J. Urol. 2003'170(2 Pt 2: S24-9

Wright, PJ. "Comparison of Phosphodiesterase Type 5 (PDE5) Inhibitors." *Int J Clin Pract.* 2006;60(8):967-975.

Yuan J, et al. "Vacuum therapy in erectile dysfunction - Science and clinical evidence." *International Journal of Impotence Research.* 2010;22:21

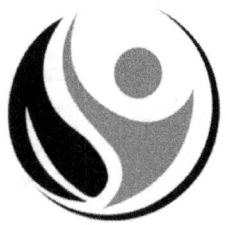

About The Authors

Mark Weis, MD is a veteran primary care physician experienced in a wide variety of clinical and leadership settings including full spectrum rural and metropolitan general practice, urgent care, emergency medicine, and medical consultant to inpatient psychiatric facilities. A national primary care thought leader who has performed numerous high level medical consulting roles for the pharmaceutical industry, Weis has been published in numerous medical journals; participated in a wide array of national continuing medical education projects; authored two novels, including the Christian crisis of faith thriller, **Lead Me Into Temptation**, and **Over The Edge**—a delightful medical comedy that provides readers a shocking and enlightening look at what really goes on at psychiatric hospitals. He has also published two golf books: **Peaceful Golf: Enjoy The Game More While Improving Your Score** and **Thank You Mrs. Murphy: Behind The Curtain At The Masters Tournament**. In addition, he, along with Douglas Ginter, co-authored the highly successful **My Hormones: A Simple Guide to Better and Longer Living**—a health and wellness book that teaches readers about the harmful health effects of hormone imbalance and how these issues can be corrected with bioidentical hormone replacement therapy.

Having played significant roles in developing numerous successful medical businesses, including Canyon Health, Dr. Weis—a featured physician in both *50 Most Positive Doctors in America* (1996) and *Positive Doctors in America* (1999)—now resides in Tucson, Arizona.

Douglas Ginter has over twenty years' experience in the health care industry. The former CEO of an FDA-licensed pharmaceutical manufacturer located in Orange, California, Ginter is CEO of multiple companies, including Prescription Headquarters, a compounding pharmacy; Physicians Professional Laboratory, a CLIA certified laboratory; and Physicians Products, a physician's management company. He is also co-creator of the Clearly Beautiful line of cosmetic products used exclusively by dermatologists and plastic surgeons.

Mr. Ginter, co-author with Dr. Weis of *My Hormones: A Simple Guide to Better and Longer Living*, is a member of American Academy of Anti-Aging Medicine, American Pharmacists Association, California Pharmacy Association, and the International Academy of Compounding Pharmacists.

www.myhormones.com
www.totalmale.com